PAINDEMIC

"*Paindemic*® is a brutally honest portrayal of our current *sick care* medical model. No other book gives you such an in-depth and thought provoking overview of how pain should be assessed and treated. Dr. Cady has truly outdone herself!"

—**Jamie L. Guyden**, M.D., Integrative Medicine Physician, Austin, Texas

"*Paindemic*® is a book equally important for people in pain, health care professionals, and health care policy-makers. If you have persisting pain, you know that you need expert knowledge of this. If you are a health professional, you know it is the most common reason for patient visits, and a huge gap in professional education. Dr. Cady provides you with evidence-based information intending to compel you to change. She clearly points to the multifaceted nature of pain, asking us all to consider the manner in which we understand pain, and the manner in which we treat people with it. Given the personal costs to 20% of our populations, and the financial cost to health care agencies and society in general, we really should be considering this a *Paindemic*®."

—**Neil Pearson**, Physical Therapist, Yoga Therapist
Clinical Assistant Professor, University of British Columbia, Canada,
www.lifeisnow.ca

"I personally face the 'have a pill' merry-go-round of the current medical model. Proactive with my care and health, I find my legitimate pain concerns tend to be dismissed until the pains become difficult to overcome; only to be offered more medicines I want to avoid. Enough! *Paindemic*® opens the discussion for changes to the current protocol of the medical system. Dr. Cady brings to the forefront the ever growing problem, as only a patient with inside information can do. She understands the constraints faced by the medical teams while bringing into focus the needs of patients. I look forward to more medical personnel joining her discussions for change."

—**Donna Grumbles**, Cancer "Thriver," Dallas, Texas

"*Paindemic*® is an enlightening and informative journey through the multifaceted aspects of pain management in today's medical environment through the eyes of a physician dedicated to the treatment of pain management. The book addresses the current environment of both medicine and insurance providing a timely and important message for all of us, whether we suffer from chronic pain or not!"

—**Jana Sanders**, Insurance Professional, Austin, Texas

"It is the most helpful and useful book about pain that I have ever seen."

—**Betty Hinds**, Biologist, Texas

"It's so refreshing to see a physician that is willing to explore alternatives to surgery and narcotic medication treatments for pain management. This is a must-read for anyone who wants to learn more about managing their pain conservatively."

—**Rebecca Osborne**, Physical Therapist, Dallas, Texas

"The book *Paindemic*® reads almost as two; a guide for health care providers and a guide for patients. On one hand, it is a very good reminder to medical professionals that not having an answer does not necessarily mean you can't help your patients. I hope this book will encourage and expedite a greater collaboration between mainstream and alternative professionals, which is just beginning to happen. On the other hand, *Paindemic*® is an excellent guide for patients to take control of their health and become active participants in their wellness. Medicine, health, and wellness care must be led by patients themselves and facilitated by the professionals from which they seek care."

—**Kerri Brooker**, Chiropractor, Winnipeg, Canada

"This book is an absolute must-read for anyone who is or has a loved one suffering from chronic pain. Dr. Cady has put together an excellent one-stop chronic pain resource that will inform, educate, and guide you in navigating today's complex healthcare system."

—**Anagha Agte** M.S., Certified Clinical Somatic Educator, Austin, Texas

"Caring for my aging Grandmother has been an interesting learning experience. Reading *Paindemic*® gave me a glimpse into the scope and magnitude of the challenges my grandmother faces when it comes to having her chronic pain issues addressed. Aging is not for the weak! Thanks to reading this book I have even more compassion for my grandmother and a greater understanding of her experience; specifically of the troubles she has faced in the medical community. Most importantly, I've been given tools and vocabulary to use in an effort to aid her in getting her basic needs met."

—**Debra Hines Hathaway**, Caretaker, Austin, Texas

"I have known Dr. Cady for many years. Her drive for learning information and empowering others has always been an admirable trait. She sets an example of what to strive for and is an inspiration to many. This book is yet another opportunity for her to help enlighten and enhance people's lives beyond those who are already lucky enough to be part of her world."

—**Sonya Gonsalves**, Veterinary Tech, "Mum" of Two, Central Coast, Australia

PAINDEMIC

A Practical and Holistic Look at Chronic Pain, the Medical System, and the antiPAIN Lifestyle

MELISSA CADY, D.O.

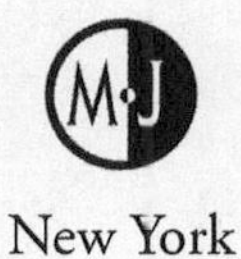

New York

PAINDEMIC

A Practical and Holistic Look at Chronic Pain, the Medical System, and the antiPAIN Lifestyle

Published in New York, New York, by Morgan James Publishing. Morgan James and The Entrepreneurial Publisher are trademarks of Morgan James, LLC.
www.MorganJamesPublishing.com

ISBN 978-1-63047-654-0 paperback
ISBN 978-1-63047-655-7 eBook
Library of Congress Control Number:
2015908194

Cover Design by:
Chris Treccani
www.3dogdesign.net

Interior Design by:
Bonnie Bushman
The Whole Caboodle Graphic Design

In Memory of Jean Jackson,
who never let Pain stand in the way of Love.

Table of Contents

A Note to the Reader

My mission is to provide the reader with an enhanced perspective and more logical approach to this country's *Paindemic*®. In doing so, I hope to steer the reader in a more practical direction to begin or change the pursuit for pain relief. However, this book is in no way establishing a patient-physician relationship. I am of the firm belief that you cannot truly evaluate, diagnose, or treat a patient without establishing a relationship with a two-way interaction. Please speak with your physician or other appropriate health care professional regarding your medical issues.

Although I reference "physicians" throughout the book, I realize there are many capable medical or health professionals who lead or influence a patient's care and may carry different titles. For the purposes of this book, the word "physician" can be used interchangeably with "medical professional" in most cases. Granted, I cannot attest to the capabilities or background of any medical practitioner, including physicians. Connecting with the right professional *for you* is part of the pain journey.

There are references and resources at the end of this book that may be of interest to you in your quest for an improved quality of life and pain relief. Since no one is exactly the same, the appropriateness of resources always *depends* on the individual.

My deepest wish for you is to find a place of less suffering, both emotionally and physically, so you can get on with your life—a life that is precious and deserves the best *from* and *for* all of us.

Foreword

by Jane C. Ballantyne, M.D.

I entered the pain field serendipitously. The work of an anesthesiologist is all about relieving pain, yet only a minority of anesthesiologists become interested in treating chronic pain. Nevertheless, early on in my personal journey, anesthesiologists pretty much owned the field of pain medicine. They were, after all, using injections and drugs to get people through surgery painlessly. Why not expand this knowledge and employ these techniques to treat pain outside the operating room? I was really only interested in pain research, but I was gradually drawn into the pain clinic. I had not experienced pain myself or been close to anyone who had suffered badly; I had no great mission to save people from pain. But it was an exciting time. The field of pain medicine had just begun, pain was designated a disease in its own right, and pain clinics were opening up everywhere. We were caught up in a fervor believing our injections and drugs could eliminate pain and make people's lives better.

Thirty years later, and what has happened? The chronic pain problem has not gone away—in fact, it has got worse. In its 2011 blueprint *Relieving Pain in America,* the Institute of Medicine (IOM) states that 116 million Americans suffer chronic pain costing up to $635 billion annually in treatment and lost productivity. "The problem of unrelieved pain remains as urgent as ever. Addressing the nation's enormous burden of pain will require a transformation in the way that pain is understood, assessed, and treated." At the same time, we are constantly reminded of the toll the nation has taken in terms of increases in opioid abuse, overdoses and deaths running parallel to increased prescribing of opioids for pain. The Centers for Disease Control (CDC) reminds us by terming the rise in prescription opioid abuse an "epidemic." The medical literature reminds us with countless new population studies warning of the dangers of overprescribing. The lay press reminds us as journalists become increasingly aware of the scandal of over-promotion by industry of expensive and risk-prone pain treatments that don't work. We live longer; we survive illnesses that not long ago were rapidly fatal, and we like to think we are healthier than ever. Then why is the pain problem getting worse and not better? What happened to all the excitement about being able to relieve people of the burden of pain through our treatments?

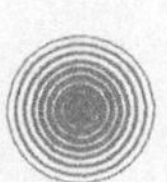

"Dr. Cady uses her book to educate patient and physician alike..."

—Jane C. Ballantyne, M.D., F.R.C.A.

Melissa Cady calls her book the *Paindemic*. She has chosen this term to embody what I have just described—the chronic pain problem getting worse and not being helped by our current treatment approach. Like me, she is an anesthesiologist with special training in pain medicine. But from there our backgrounds diverge. I learned in the school of allopathic medicine with its focus on the biophysical; she learned in the school of osteopathic medicine with its focus on mind-body and movement. I entered the field when it was a clean slate. She entered the field when we were all beginning to understand the limits of allopathic medicine. When we see patients in pain clinics nowadays, it is rare that we see patients who have not already started on the pain journey; more often, we see patients who have been on the journey for years, and they are in trouble. We see the problems of overreliance on "miracle cures," lack of acceptance of pain, and lack of engagement in the process of self-management. We have learned the importance of what often seems elusive, a healthy lifestyle, a key factor in managing pain well. Dr. Cady uses her book to educate patient and physician alike, on why we develop chronic pain, when chronic pain needs medical intervention and when not, what the proper role for medical treatments is, where complementary approaches can help, and most important of all, what we can do for ourselves. What she stresses throughout her book is that we can no longer afford to take a passive role and wait for something or someone to come along and take the pain away. Active engagement in the process of becoming healthy will do more to rid us of chronic pain than anything else. Understanding this and incorporating it into our lives is the cultural change the IOM is crying out for, and Dr. Cady's book is an invaluable step toward achieving it.

—**Jane C. Ballantyne**, M.D., F.R.C.A.
President of PROP (Physicians for Responsible Opioid Prescribing)
Professor, Anesthesiology and Pain Medicine, University of Washington

Preface

If you have pain or know someone with pain, you may be comforted to know that I have dealt with pain, too. My journey began in my late twenties while I was in medical school. I was very active and training others to be active. One day, while pushing a heavy weight with one leg, I felt a twinge in the lower right area of my back. Like so many others who experience pain, I did not have severe pain at the time of the likely cause of injury. The next day was a different story! I had pain that was so exquisite and debilitating; I could not bend over and tie my shoes for six months! The first doctor I saw was an osteopathic physician (D.O.) who told me not to do any exercise for two weeks. I didn't feel like this was the right course of action, but it was what the doctor recommended—and he knows more than I do, right? Well, I was worse after two weeks. I was also confused, and I was in medical school! Anatomy classes are one thing. Yet, just because you ace an anatomy course does not mean you know how the mechanics of the human body really work nor pain in general. Fortunately, being in the osteopathic medical school program gave me some insight and, more importantly, a vigilance to find some answers.

As can be expected, the low back pain did not self-resolve after being *less active* for two weeks. After four more opinions from a second D.O. and three

M.D.s, I was frustrated. Fortunately, one of my fellow medical students invited me to a class to learn how to treat musculoskeletal issues. Her father, who also happened to be an osteopathic physician, led the training. It turned out I was one of the guinea pigs for the discussion and hands-on tutorial. He recognized my asymmetries and tension and performed a significant amount of deep tissue release on the connective tissue. Within twenty minutes, I stood up from the table with most of my pain gone and a greater range of motion than I had experienced in weeks! Over the course of the following year, I was able to go from experiencing residual pain to being pain-free. Happily, the most invasive treatment I had to undergo was an X-ray of my previously painful yet *normal* left hip. I was able to avoid injections, opioids, and surgery—thank goodness! I consider myself one of the lucky ones. I truly believe everyone should have the best chance of relieving or avoiding pain without extreme risk. It should not just be for the lucky!

As a physician, I have witnessed patients making difficult, sometimes almost unfathomable decisions regarding treatment for their pain. The sheer desperation and confusion I've seen firsthand from my friends, family, colleagues, and patients who are in pain have substantiated my belief that a complex medical web has developed which may be causing, perpetuating, exploiting, or exacerbating a patient's pain. Yet, only a small percentage actually gets better.

Helping someone in pain is not as straightforward as other problems, such as cataracts, which are easier to diagnose and treat. **Pain can be elusive. Pain can be difficult to categorize. Pain can be hard to manage. Chronic pain can leave the patient, and physician, feeling frustrated and hopeless.**

It is difficult to choose among the array of assessment and treatment options available to pain patients and their physicians. Even my colleagues are confused about where to start or go for help with their own pain. It seems crazy that they are not sure where to begin—they are in the medical community! In truth, the solutions presented to patients suffering from chronic pain are based on and limited to the opinions of the provider or providers chosen. Therefore, it is no surprise that patients may not be fully informed of *all* the options available. Even *reputable* physicians have been known to *sell* treatments to patients that may or may not be necessary, leading patients to opt for riskier procedures or strong, possibly addicting, medications. Yet, most physicians have their hearts in the right place and care about their patients.

In spite of good intentions, physicians are caught in the world of "insurance reimbursement," which pays for riskier, more expensive procedures, but pays little or nothing for less invasive treatments, including education. Physicians, especially those just trying to become established, would have a difficult time surviving, paying their heavy debts, or reaching their fiscal expectations in their practice if they recommended more noninvasive approaches *versus* lucrative or readily reimbursed procedures. Physicians must play the game of jumping through the insurance hoops just to get patients approved for helpful, or sometimes not so helpful, services.

There are many choices out there for pain management: pills, injections, surgeries, and a barrage of technological advances. Yet, there is a deficit of helpful education for pain patients regarding how to listen to the body and how to use less invasive approaches to improve or relieve pain. Ignoring this and only offering riskier alternatives is as silly as offering gastric bypass surgery for every person who wants to lose weight. Weight can be lost, but it may not be the best way to shed excess pounds. Gastric bypass surgery comes with a higher price tag, anesthetic risks, and increased nutritional health concerns due to the permanent alteration of the body. Unfortunately, many patients who undergo surgery learn about the side effects or complications of their procedure afterward.

The availability of fancy and technically advanced options does not mean these are the only or *best* way of going about treating a pain problem. They are simply marketed more heavily and appear to be a quick or passive "fix" for something that could be dealt with in a more natural and healthier way. Sadly, many of these options are pushed in the name of not just profit, but greed. Greed is a contributor to the inflation of health care costs, attributable to the "medical middlemen," such as hospitals, insurance companies, medical device companies, and pharmaceutical companies. The depth and breadth of the negative influences of political and regulatory involvement is beyond the scope of this book, but truly complicate this pain epidemic even further. With so many forces working against patients, it can be easy for a patient to "punt" and take the easiest route even if it means lifelong medication or potential surgical complications.

Despite the fact that I am a doctor of osteopathic medicine, I don't think I would have understood the struggles of being a pain patient if I had not gone through it myself. Knowing that patients can avoid drugs, injections, and surgery and still may experience 100 percent relief, as I did, is what drove me to write this book. I occasionally have recurrences of pain, which I have been able to easily manage for the last 15 years.

It is this experience and the noninvasive treatments I used to reclaim my life and eliminate my pain that I wish to share. Regardless how the chronic pain began, optimizing health can only make things better. It all starts by listening to the body and understanding what it needs. It also starts by understanding the other alternatives available beyond the current practice of opioids, injections, and surgery.

More importantly, I believe most pain patients are willing and capable of leading an antiPAIN Lifestyle! I am here to give a practical perspective and empower those who want to avoid being a statistic in this country's PAINDEMIC®! Join me, a physician-turned-patient, on the journey to managing and overcoming chronic pain using methods that are healthy, sustainable, and nearly risk-free. What have you got to lose…except chronic pain?

PART 1

THE PAIN PROBLEM

CHAPTER 1

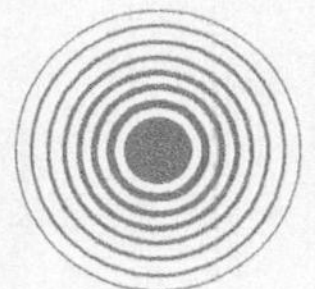

Paindemic®: There is Pain Everywhere!

Behind every beautiful thing, there's some kind of pain.
—Bob Dylan

Pain is everywhere and part of the human experience. An estimate in 2011 showed that over 100 million Americans suffer from some type of chronic pain, and a percentage of those have *severe and disabling* chronic pain. That number exceeds the number of Americans with diabetes, heart disease, or cancer combined. The annual cost estimate at that time was more than $600 billion dollars in terms of direct medical expenses and lost productivity. It is safe to say that the number keeps climbing.[1]

The profusion of pain statistics is shocking, especially stats for *low back pain—one of the most common pain complaints today*. The title of this book underscores pain's pervasiveness in our society and is a play on the word *pandemic*, which means occurring over a wide geographic area and affecting a high proportion of the population. **A *Paindemic*® is an epidemic (or pandemic) of chronic pain and the associated overutilization of pills, injections, and surgeries**. This overutilization has led to some dire and unintended consequences. Unfortunately, pain isn't simply a problem in the U.S.

Among 21 regions of the world in the Global Burden of Disease Study of 2010, low back pain was *one of the top four* common disorders out of 289 disabling conditions. In all *developed* countries, low back pain took the number one place in terms of length of time suffering. Sadly, this statistic has not changed substantially since 1990.[2] Closer to home, a 2011 U.S. Gallup poll found that out of approximately 350,000 adult Americans, 47 percent had some type of chronic pain while 31 percent of them specifically had neck or back pain.[3]

Because there is such a wide variety of pain experience, it may be helpful to define pain more concretely. Per the International Association for the Study of Pain:

> **Pain is an unpleasant sensory and emotional experience associated with actual or potential tissue damage, or described in terms of such damage.**[4]

In general, the two types of pain are:

1. **Nociceptive**: pain that arises from actual or threatened damage to *non-nerve* tissue. A paper cut to the skin is an example of an experience of *nociceptive* pain.
2. **Neuropathic**: pain caused by a disease or injury to the *nervous system*.
   a. *Central neuropathic pain* relates to the brain and spinal cord. Central pain occurs as a response to many disorders, diseases, and traumas including multiple sclerosis and strokes. Stroke victims can complain of pain or burning on the side affected by the stroke. A prime example of central pain is the phantom pain often experienced by amputees. In phantom pain, the amputee may feel real pain in the missing body part; however, the reported pain is perceived centrally, or in the brain.

b. *Peripheral neuropathic pain* is related to damage to nerves beyond the brain and spinal cord. It could be related to damage from diabetes, chemotherapy drugs, infections, or trauma. Pain from carpal tunnel syndrome is an example of peripheral neuropathic pain.

Pain serves to enhance human survival. It alerts the brain of a potential threat, which triggers a response. In the case of touching a hot stove, the triggered response is a quick pulling back and, perhaps, a loud, "Ouch!" It is NOT a specific "pain message." Different receptors such as those sensing temperature or pressure deliver information or *stimuli* through pathways to the spinal cord and brain. The brain then *interprets* that stimuli as a *painful experience*; thereby leading to pulling back from the hot stove. Yet, all of this happens so fast that humans cannot sense these multiple steps.

Pain is one of the few areas of medicine where there is *not* much objective evidence to prove a patient is experiencing pain. Inherent assumptions are typically made by nearby observers. For example, if a woman in labor is crying out during contractions, nearby observers would all agree that she is experiencing pain. In fact, the experience of acute pain is typically reflected in a rising heart rate and blood pressure. Pain is, however, more frequently *endured*, that is, the pain exists, but no screaming announces its presence. Pain is part of the normal human existence, and almost everyone experiences it. For those who *cannot* feel pain, they are born with a rare mutation, which can lead to negative consequences, such as breaking a leg or burning skin without any alert from the body's sensors. For those who can feel pain and are suffering from chronic pain, the pain experience never ends. The presence of pain affects all aspects of life—mental, physical, and emotional.

People experience pain based on their unique nervous system or "wiring," and how individuals deal with pain varies. Some people tolerate mental and physical stresses without complaint, but others are extremely affected and often very expressive about their stress. Life experiences can also dictate how pain is managed, and the degree to which it is tolerated can change over time. In fact, research supports the phenomenon of *neuroplasticity,* meaning the brain is always adapting and changing based on life events.

Neuroplasticity is the property of the brain that enables it to change its own structure and functioning in response to activity and mental experience.[5]

Pain is identified in two ways: acute or chronic.

1. **Acute** pain is fleeting and resolves within a specific timeframe. A paper cut, bruise, slight burn, or twisted ankle may hurt for hours, days, or weeks but typically resolves within three to six months. Much of this depends on the body's unique ability to heal. If the acute pain does not diminish, it can become chronic.
2. **Chronic** pain can suddenly appear and may have no easily defined cause. The pain can be intense and restrict movement, which can persist if not treated. By definition, chronic pain does not self-resolve, meaning sufferers must follow a treatment regimen to improve function and reduce the pain. Chronic pain is the primary focus of this book.

In general, pain is an *experience* due to harmful or unpleasant stimuli triggering a cascade of events affecting and interacting with the brain. With chronic pain, those events repeatedly happen and allow the pain to persist, which can be distracting and frustrating. There are three basic ways to deal with chronic pain: pinpoint the cause, mask the symptoms, or ignore it. While it can be challenging to identify, locating or pinpointing the cause of the pain makes the most sense intuitively. However, it is common for physicians to recommend masking the symptoms of pain or recommend treatments that *might* fix the problem. In my opinion, pain should never be ignored or masked, except for brief periods of time or only as a last resort.

Living with long-term pain can have serious consequences for the nervous system. Due to neuroplasticity, chronic pain can lead to *sensitization.* This sensitization can develop into an *increased* response to harmful or unpleasant stimuli, known as *hyperalgesia.* This hypersensitivity can be so extreme that it can make a person experience pain when touched by something typically *non-painful.* This condition is called *allodynia.* For example, draping a thin sheet over a pain sufferer's feet can be excruciatingly painful *if allodynia is present.*[6,7]

Red Flags

As noted above, pain serves to indicate something is amiss in the body. Determining whether the problem is acutely threatening is the first priority. In other words, what are the *red flags* that could be suggesting a real threat?

Pain is not usually deadly, although it can add stress to an already compromised system such as someone with heart disease. **Pain itself is the central nervous system's interpretation or alert that there is a problem.** In addition to pain, there may be other signs or symptoms to indicate an urgent or emergent situation.

Some of the *Alarming Signs and Symptoms* that could be related to pain include, but are not limited to:

- Throwing up blood
- Trouble swallowing
- Rectal bleeding
- Blood in urine
- Loss of strength or feeling in arm(s) or leg(s)
- Loss of control of urinating or defecating
- Unexpected, significant weight loss

Some of the *rare* conditions that could be associated with pain (especially with the back) include, but are not limited to:

- Cancer
- Infection
- Spinal osteomyelitis
- Spinal fracture
- Cauda equina syndrome
- Dissecting/ruptured aortic aneurysm
- Arachnoiditis

Much of the pain people endure is not life-threatening, but it can be life changing and sometimes lifelong if approached inappropriately. If pain is present, it is best to have a physician do a *thorough* history and physical to eliminate or uncover serious issues. Determining those issues and pinpointing the cause of the pain is not always easy.

The human body is not always straightforward, and the nervous system is not a simple or direct highway. For example, a person suffering from heart disease may be experiencing pain in the left arm but not in the chest area. This type of *referred pain* means the brain is *perceiving* the pain at a location other than the site of the painful stimulus. Although the pain is *perceived* in the arm, the heart is the underlying problem. There are many proposed explanations for referred pain, but in essence, the brain is receiving information or stimuli and *trying to make the most sense of the perceived problem*. The brain may then project pain in an area of the body unrelated to the issue; thus, it is not always perfect at mapping.[8]

The nervous system is like a confusing array of innumerable highway intersections accompanied by varied interpretations. Thus, the nerves have unique ways of influencing certain symptoms. This complexity can undermine "the best guess" as to the underlying problem, which is why it is better to enlist the help of a physician to **rule out red flags**. Truthfully, even in the absence of obvious symptoms, it is wise to see a physician to be certain nothing serious is going on.

All chronic pain began as acute pain; therefore, acute pain is just as important as chronic pain. **Unresolved acute pain, left untreated or treated improperly, stands a much greater chance of becoming chronic pain**. In the U.S. and other developed nations, the number of individuals living with chronic pain continues to increase—this is truly a *Paindemic*. Because of these numbers, chronic pain has become big business, and this is not necessarily in the best interests of chronic pain sufferers.

CHAPTER 2

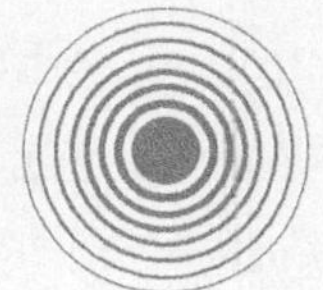

Humans Don't Come with a Manual at Birth

Until man duplicates a blade of grass, nature can laugh at his so-called scientific knowledge. Remedies from chemicals will never stand in favor compared with the products of nature, the living cell of the plant, the final result of the rays of the sun, the mother of all life.

—Thomas Edison

The human body is a miraculous bit of machinery, not unlike today's cars. Cars typically come with a manual or a troubleshooting guide in the event there are problems or for maintenance guidance. At some point, the car may develop a noise, a leak, or have a part fail. Sometimes the fix is straightforward, but sometimes mechanics have trouble figuring out the problem. Occasionally, the so-called "fix" may not address the real cause but merely reduce the symptoms; hence, the problem was not resolved. Even though humans wrote the car repair manual, it often takes time, observation, and troubleshooting to decipher problems. Compared to the human body, cars are easy to fix. Humans, unfortunately, don't come with a manual and are *not* put together like a car.

The human body is miraculous, complex, and intricately designed. Simple solutions to complex problems rarely exist. Two people presenting with the same symptoms could have very different issues underlying those symptoms. The human body is complicated. It is for this reason research and multiple opinions about the human body exist. With all of the centuries of human study, scientists, researchers, and physicians still do not know everything there is to know. In the study and research of medicine, clinicians tend to use specific terms to reflect the extent of human understanding, or lack thereof. These descriptive terms include:

- *unclear*
- *maybe*
- *could*
- *possibly*
- *sometimes*
- *typically*
- *unknown*
- *uncertainty*
- *limited knowledge*
- *theory*

New medical advances are being made every day, and much is still awaiting discovery.

Physicians spend years in school and then in residency to become highly skilled, but that does not mean everything they were taught is accurate or appropriate for patients. Many people assume physicians understand everything about the body. As a rule, physicians take great pride in what they do know and find it incredibly difficult *not* to know something. It is ingrained in their training—*to know.*

In a recent article, the well-published Dr. David Katz frankly stated:

I don't know the answer, but it shakes my faith. In science, we know darn well that we are missing data. Science is the struggle to know truths that are subtle, and at times stubbornly elusive. The only way to them is incremental, accelerated by the occasional epiphany courtesy of rare genius. Scientific truth comes together slowly, and along the way is riddled with fenestrations.[9]

In my opinion, those "fenestrations" or gaps are the essence of this book and the reason for the *Paindemic*. For if we understood *pain* more clearly, then we could manage it better.

The basis for physicians to acquire their degree is centered on their *knowledge*. When confronted by something *unknown*, they may feel uncomfortable. Not knowing is hard on a physician's ego, especially when a patient is relying on the physician's answers for pain relief and the physician is genuinely trying to help. For that reason, when things do not make sense, it is common for *some* physicians to assume their patients are being difficult or unfortunately a little crazy.

Thankfully, not all physicians think this way. However, even well-intentioned physicians may inadvertently harm their patients in an effort to help. These big-hearted physicians may try procedures or medications to see if they *happen* to work. When the procedures or treatments fail to perform as hoped, physicians face the reality that *there is a limit to their knowledge of the human body* despite many advances. Fortunately, most physicians accept that they are forever *students* of medicine, as there is an art and evolution to medical knowledge. Chronic pain is one such area that remains largely a mystery, even though extensive research has been conducted. According to pain expert, Dr. Steven King, "To say the medical community's knowledge of chronic pain is scant is something of an understatement."[10]

As humans, physicians can fall victim to adhering too tightly to specific knowledge without considering other possible options or courses of treatment. In the world of pain medicine, this frequently occurs. When some physicians are presented with options outside traditional training to help others in pain, it is not unusual for them to scoff, disbelieve, or even discredit the methods. I know—I have done it myself. *Sometimes physicians need the burden of proof before believing or recommending a therapy.* These physicians operate under the assumption, if it wasn't taught in medical training or read in well-supported research, then it is irrelevant or cannot be recommended.

A case in point involves Dr. Caldwell Esselstyn, a *surgeon* who has shown amazing results for reversing and preventing heart disease with a *plant-based food lifestyle.*[11] While the results are beyond promising for heart disease sufferers, little effort is made by most cardiologists or other physicians to educate and advise patients (especially those who are at high risk for heart attacks) to adopt this type of diet.[12] There is a cost for not educating patients. By not sharing this dietary advice, physicians potentially doom their patients to an over $100,000 price tag for a heart bypass surgery or worse, contribute to the progression of heart disease, heart attack, or death.

Not all physicians downplay new discoveries and alternative options, thankfully. As some begin to recognize their limitations in their education and training, they seek out more information on their own. For example, their acceptance of differing treatment options is enhanced when the physician becomes a patient dealing with chronic pain. Then, the gaps in the medical community's collective knowledge are obvious, and they see firsthand the medical system's inadequacies, sometimes discovering better ways to approach the issue.

Understanding physician knowledge gaps is important because some may not value the same things presented in this book, not because physicians do not care, but because they have not been taught or gained an appreciation for these solutions. I do not claim to know everything about what I emphasize, but I do know that what has helped me is *outside the scope of most traditional medical training programs.* The physician's focus should be to help patients improve. However, it is also up to the patient to engage in a discussion of *all* treatment options to find a workable and personalized solution.

Physicians are human, and patients should not be intimidated to respectfully communicate with their physicians. If patients do not understand or do not like how they have been treated, then they should speak up. Granted, some patients' expectations are more reasonable than others while some patients are perfectly content with being passive in their medical care and lives. Just like children who get their way with unhealthy fast-food meals from their parents, their health over the long run suffers when they are not taught better life skills. The former is quick and easy, but the latter takes time and education. A physician's goal is to do what is best for a patient's health, not solely to make a patient happy. Usually *healthy* patients are *happy* patients, but getting to "healthy" is not always a happy process. The more physicians are challenged by patients who advocate their health, the more physicians will learn, thus enabling them to help other patients in similar circumstances.

It is easy to use a car as an analogy for the human body. But humans are NOT cars; the body is much more complex than a Volvo or Chevy. Just as finding the right mechanic for a particular make of car ensures the right knowledge to fix that car, finding the right physician who understands and seeks a variety of solutions to a problem ensures a wider field of treatments and procedures. This creates great potential for avoiding high-risk, high-cost "fixes." Physicians are only as good as their knowledge, compassion, and curiosity, which can be extraordinarily helpful. Yet, patients must be advocates for their own health, as well, not simply taking what a physician says as "gospel." After all, humans are born with a placenta, not a manual.

CHAPTER 3

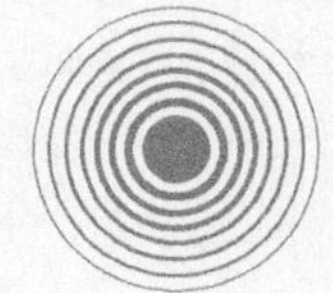

The Invisible Burden: Out of Sight or *Out of Your Mind*?

Pain is strange. A cat killing a bird, a car accident, a fire...Pain arrives, BANG, and there it is, it sits on you. It's real. And to anybody watching, you look foolish. Like you've suddenly become an idiot. There's no cure for it unless you know somebody who understands how you feel, and knows how to help.

—**Charles Bukowski**, American Author

To the outside observer, a pain sufferer might appear a little nuts. The patient may seem perfectly fine, but be in a constant state of torment. Crankiness, a short temper, unexpected crying jags—the emotions behind pain can be varied and unpredictable. Coupling those emotions with not being believed can push pain patients over the edge. They might even begin to believe they are crazy. Per the International Association for the Study of Pain (IASP):

> *...Pain is always subjective...always unpleasant and therefore also an emotional experience... There is usually no way to distinguish their experience from that due to tissue damage if we take the subjective report... it should be accepted as pain...pain, which is always a psychological state, even though we may well appreciate that pain most often has a proximate [immediate] physical cause.*[13]

In other words, for a pain sufferer, the best thing they can hear is, "I believe you." Ironically, when a patient does not feel believed, it could actually *worsen* the pain.

Physicians must trust the patient is telling the truth, even though there are those *rare* individuals who may have an ulterior motive for becoming a patient. Ultimately, physicians cannot *experience* a patient's *physical* pain, just as they cannot *experience* a patient's *emotional* pain. Both are *pain* as experienced by the brain. Whereas the physical manifestations of emotional pain, such as crying, are accepted by observers, it is harder to understand someone's pain when there is no physical cue such as with a headache or backache. This can be in stark contrast to an obviously broken bone; suffering is expected. Without visual verification, physicians can struggle to verify, identify, or quantify pain.

Pain's invisibility also creates roadblocks to discovering its cause. Unlike a broken bone, pain may not be so clear-cut. Because of pain's elusive nature and the discomfort of dealing with the unknown, physicians often have a difficult time empathizing with the pain patient. This lack of empathy can sideline the doctor-patient relationship since the patient may not feel heard or understood by the one person from which the patient needs the most help.

One such pain complaint is complex regional pain syndrome (CRPS), previously known as reflex sympathetic dystrophy. CRPS can present in a variety of ways, for example, a minor foot injury can progress to *burning pain when a normally pleasurable touch occurs* (aka allodynia). This injury can lead to pain in other areas of the body as well. For physicians unsure of the CRPS diagnosis or are biased against it, the patient can be labeled as drug-seeking, attention-seeking, or worse. When physicians cannot prove what is going on with a patient, they may feel compelled to give an explanation based on what they have been taught or at least assign a reasonable diagnosis. Unfortunately, under these circumstances, those diagnoses can be wrong or unhelpful.

Without visual confirmation, it can become uncomfortable and frustrating for the physician and the patient to seek the answer or cause of pain. As difficult as it is, physicians need to become comfortable with being occasionally stumped by a patient's symptoms. It may take some time and exploration. Regardless, medical clinicians should try to empathize with the patient's plight and find other providers or methods to assist the patient in deciphering the cause and symptoms of the pain. At the same time, the patient needs to be aware of and have patience with the process of discovery.

Classic medical history provides an uncomfortable example of how knowing versus not knowing the answers for a patient's condition can color the perspective or affect the treatment of a patient. Within the last 200 years, seizures in children were interpreted as the child being possessed by an evil spirit, demon, or the devil. Today, we understand seizures to be brain issues, not the work of evil spirits.

Physicians don't always have answers, but that is the beauty of the patient and physician working together and digging deeper to understand the patient's dilemma. In those cases, it may require a multi-provider or inter-disciplinary effort to get a broader or more focused evaluation of the patient's issue. It may also take a collaborative effort between the patient and physician to battle the medical intermediaries or "middlemen" (e.g., health insurance) that may be hindering ideal care.

When doctors become patients due to pain, the lack of knowledge and help from their medical counterparts can be the cause for profound dismay and frustration. Below is a real-life account of a physician-patient, Dr. Joy Whipple, who underwent an evaluation of post-surgical, scar-related disease.

> *I have been startled to find myself on the other end as a patient and the frank lack of dignity this [pain] population must endure...I am familiar with the blank stares from medical professionals but am fortunate to have the educational capacity to help myself. What does work is what you can do*

rather than what you can't, regardless of the ongoing medical focus dictated by an insurance-driven industry.[14]

Physicians owe it to patients to keep an open mind and truly listen, so they have a better perspective of the patient's pain experience. Some of the biggest complaints from patients about their physicians are that they do not feel heard or their symptoms are minimized.

We must remember that what we know now in medicine may be considered false in the future; the opposite is also true. The physician and the patient should understand there are opportunities for learning on both sides, but clinicians must be humble enough to understand their limitations. In the end, physicians must always listen to the patient. In the world of insurance with high-volume practices, there is little time to do what the patient and the physician need most: listening and communicating. The erosion of an effective patient-physician relationship has no place when dealing with chronic pain. Worst of all, dismissing the patient's pain is as devastating as crushing a patient's hope. **It is the "patient," not the physician, who experiences a patient's pain.**

CHAPTER 4

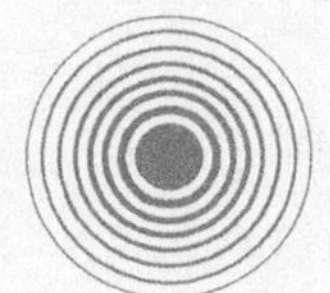

Your Body's Ability to Adapt and Heal

Instead of seeing the body as a machine that, like a new car, must deteriorate over time, we should see it as a system that learns, adapts, and improves over time.

—**Deepak Chopra, M.D.**

The human body inherently favors balance or *homeostasis*. Homeostasis is the tendency toward a relatively stable equilibrium. This happens in many ways, such as the acid-alkaline balance, which has a pH value *around* 7.35 to 7.45 in living, healthy humans. Significant variations from this range are incompatible with human life. Temperature regulation is another area. No conscious thought goes into regulating pH, body temperature or any other automatic processes the human body does to keep it in balance. A body in balance is a happy body. When the body is stressed, imbalance occurs, which can set the stage for illness, injury, or other chronic problems.

Bad habits are frequently the reason the human body is pushed out of balance such as excessive alcohol consumption, constant sitting, lack of physical activity, smoking, inadequate water intake, eating processed food, inadequate sleep, or persistently high stress environments. Other stressors may include some prescription drugs or verbal abuse.

Those bad habits or stressors can bring out the worst from a human's genes. For example, a person with a family history of high blood pressure and obesity does not necessarily resign that person to developing those health issues. There may be a genetic predisposition, but in most cases, a clean diet and adequate exercise may be just the thing to prevent that person from becoming another family health statistic. However, if the susceptible genetics and healthy habits are ignored, the person could end up imbalanced and, like other family members, obese and on high blood pressure medication.

The point is this: *genetics is only one part of the equation*. Just because members of a family have debilitating back pain does not necessarily mean *all* family members are destined for back pain. Many decisions are made every day leading to behaviors and habits, which ultimately influence health. The human body is constantly striking a balance between genetics and lifestyle. In other words, an individual's susceptibilities or vulnerabilities (*genetics*) are at the mercy of that person's daily habits or insults (*lifestyle*). By making better choices most of the time, the patient is allowing the body to be better equipped at warding off problems or disorders. Also by making better choices, the body can remain in its favored state—balance.

The effects of daily habits may be difficult to see and even harder to accept. As an example, obstructive sleep apnea diagnosed in later life does not show up overnight. In *most* cases, visible excess weight gain is the primary contributor and takes months, years, or decades to develop. Each body type and airway is different, but there is a tipping point of weight gain whereby the soft tissues and accumulated fat in the neck relax and compress the airway during deep sleep. This imbalance can be life-threatening.

Sometimes more extreme examples, which emphasize the cumulative effect of small changes or choices over time, are necessary to bring the point home. Below are two illustrations of the incredible adaptability of human beings.

The Olympic Runner

Suppose an Olympic runner ended up in the intensive care unit after a car accident with a broken leg. For every day the leg is immobilized, the patient's strength decreases by 1 to 1.5 percent per day. After five weeks of total inactivity, muscle strength is reduced by 50 percent! If no muscle contraction occurs in the leg, its strength eventually plummets to 25 to 40 percent of the runner's original strength. Because of inactivity and lack of muscle pulling on the bone, osteopenia could also occur, leaching added calcium from the bone into the bloodstream. This could lead to an elevated calcium level known as hypercalcemia. All of these could be avoided by doing one simple thing daily: one leg muscle contraction at 50 percent of the runner's maximal strength. This slight "exercise" would be enough to prevent the additional loss of strength from the inactive leg.[15]

Inactivity, which can also mean minimal or low workloads, does not only affect the muscles; it can increase the heart rate approximately 0.5 beats per minute per day. This phenomenon is *immobilization tachycardia*. In addition, the amount of blood pumped by the heart can decrease by 15 percent after only two weeks of bed rest due to blood volume changes and blood pooling in the leg veins. Most people would recognize that an Olympic runner subjected to five weeks of bed rest would not be able to run as before without slowly working back up to that level. In fact, standing and walking would be the first challenge for the runner to do successfully. In other words, the human body makes changes incrementally based on what *is* done or *not* done.[16]

The Astronaut

Gravity not only keeps people and things grounded on the earth, it also provides a daily gentle stressor that, for living beings, encourages some muscle tone. The weightless atmosphere experienced by astronauts in space is a different story. Upon returning to Earth from long space flights, it is normal for astronauts to be weak and have difficulty standing or walking. In fact, aerospace specialists have reported that while the typical earth-bound adult human loses 1 to 2 percent of their muscle mass over ten years; an astronaut loses that same amount of muscle mass in one month in space! Evidently, the challenge of gravity is of great benefit to humans.[17]

There are other issues for astronauts beyond muscle tone. A sustained weightless environment such as an extended space flight to Mars could see astronauts losing bone density at astronomical (no pun intended) speeds. It could be the equivalent to bone loss over a lifetime on Earth. This loss increases the risk of fractures, promotes overall weakness and the development of painful urinary stones. Exercise in space helps slow down bone loss, but it could still take almost two years of training upon returning to Earth to compensate for the loss. The adage, "use it or lose it," is quite apt for the human body in space.[18]

Back on Earth, sometimes the body's impressive ability to adapt may lead to *dysfunction* in a location of the body unrelated to the cause or problem, as can happen after a broken leg. At first, crutches may be required to get around

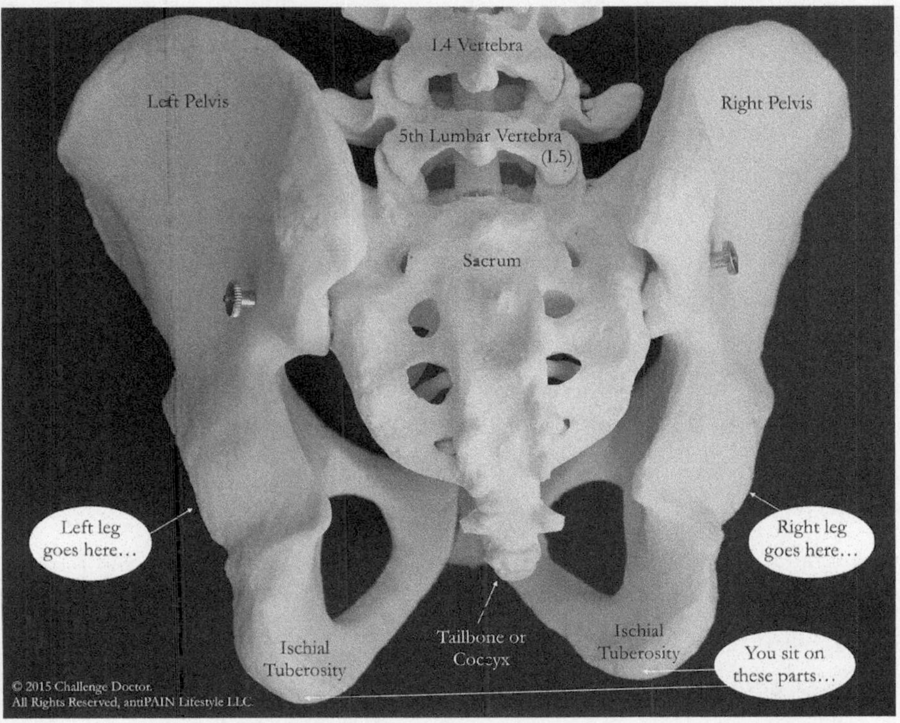

Figure 1: The sacrum and each side of the pelvis are shown here. Don't be fooled. Bones are not the only thing affected by changes in the human body's movements—ligaments, tendons, muscles, and other connective tissues are affected too.

without putting pressure on the broken leg. Next, a walking cast or a special boot allows pressure to be placed on the injured leg when walking. It is not uncommon at this point for people with legs healing in casts to complain of low back pain—sometimes even after the cast or boot is removed. Yet, frequently, no low back pain was present before the broken leg happened. The pain perceived in the back could occur from alterations in the gait, which could be from several factors including the weight of the boot or the leg being pushed upward due to the thick boot sole.

Humans have two legs, two sides to the pelvis, but only *one* spine. (see Figure 1) The spine, which includes the sacrum, is suspended by an enormous number of connections between the two sides of the pelvis. The optimum state for the spine is neutral—balanced equally between the two sides. When a leg is broken, the body naturally accommodates the injury by adjusting the pelvis, spine, and legs to allow walking. This adaptation could cause the spine to adjust away from neutral creating more chance for pain to be perceived in the low back, pelvis, or leg.

A broken leg can heal. For a leg amputee, the imbalance is forever—even if the person uses a prosthetic device. A prosthetic leg enables the amputee to live a normal life, almost as if the leg was still present. Prosthetic legs, for all the advances, still cannot perfectly imitate a human leg. Although typically subtle, a gait adjustment happens because the prosthetic leg has a less elegant motion compared to a normally functioning leg. Leg amputees commonly complain of back pain. This can be caused by a variety of factors including poor prosthetic fit and alignment, postural changes, leg-length discrepancy, amputation level, or general deconditioning. Creating further problems, the load that an amputee places on the intact leg is greater than the force someone without an amputation would exert on legs during natural walking. Hence, joint pain or problems frequently occur in an amputee's intact leg.[19]

The more drastic the leg amputation, the more likely the amputee will have pain problems. In a study, above-knee amputees were more likely to have back pain (81 percent) than below-knee amputees (63 percent). In addition, overweight amputees were more likely to have back pain. The study also found that 63 percent of amputees experienced moderate to severe back pain and 60 percent had back pain that *started within two years* after amputation. Remarkably, MRI scan findings did NOT show degenerative arthritis-related asymmetries, suggesting *functional imbalances* were causing pain.[20] The takeaway is that alterations in the body's structure or function can *immediately or slowly* start affecting the balance of human bodies, and *possibly* lead to pain. Asymmetries are not strictly isolated to the domain of amputees; everyone has them. Some of them are just harder to spot with intact bodies, especially by untrained eyes. Whether that asymmetry is relevant to pain is another challenge to unravel, because perceived asymmetries do not always correlate with problems or pain.

Aside from what can be seen, there are ongoing, *invisible* changes to genes that are reacting to a human's behavior and environment. Unfavorable insults such as poor nutrition or injuries to the human body can accumulate over time and can directly affect its genes. It may not be obvious at first, but the genetic vulnerability is eventually unveiled such as in many chronic diseases. Although a change in gene *expression* does not affect the actual inherited DNA *sequence* for that person, the altered expression can affect the generations that follow. In other words, the genes each person are born with are influenced by their parents' previous behavior, the environment, and personal habits. In the context of chronic pain, one example is traumatic childhood stressors, which can alter gene expression and increase pain sensitivity. The human body, including its genes, intuitively responds to everything done *by* or *to* the body, whether it is consciously aware of it or not. This phenomenon is called *epigenetics* and is a new area of research.[21]

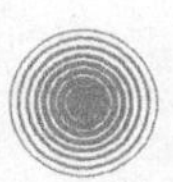

"Humans can underestimate positive yet subtle changes occurring from beneficial lifestyle choices; consequently, they frequently quit too soon to see the potentially worthwhile manifestations."

Whether invisible or visible to the naked eye, changes from the genes to the skin occur without conscious awareness. For that reason, humans can underestimate positive yet subtle changes occurring from beneficial lifestyle choices; consequently, they frequently quit too soon to see the potentially worthwhile manifestations. Equally threatening is the denial of subtle negative changes that can occur from unhealthy behaviors. **The bottom line is that the human body is incredibly complex with an inherent intelligence to adapt and heal itself. Choosing poor habits and lifestyle can push the body out of balance, potentially leading to new or more pain**.

CHAPTER 5

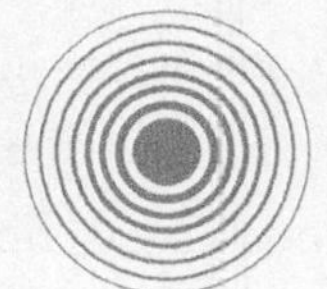

The Dilemma of Pain Avoidance

We are more often frightened than hurt; and we suffer more from imagination than from reality.

—**Lucius Annaeus Seneca**, Roman Philosopher

The body can adapt to many insults or patterns, whether that adaptation is beneficial or not. When pain occurs and does not continue to improve, it is defined as *chronic*. There is no specific point when pain changes from acute to chronic; it depends upon the individual's healing process and other factors. Professionals often use a three-month or six-month timeline to categorize pain as chronic, but healing rates vary based on the injury. The definition is less important than the *response to pain*. Commonly, activities are altered or stopped to avoid the pain. Unless a person is healing after a bone fracture or other form of trauma such as surgery, the tendency to minimize or eliminate pain by avoiding normal activity or movement can often make the pain worse.

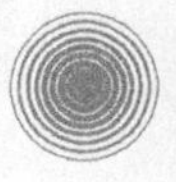

"...the tendency to minimize or eliminate pain by avoiding normal activity or movement can often make the pain worse."

The **human body is meant to move**; therefore, there is no benefit to restricting or limiting motion. Many times, avoidance of pain decreases involvement with others or participating in favorite activities. This withdrawal becomes the breeding ground for depression if the isolation continues. The pain itself can become a fixation, and as the pain continues, more physical and psychological adaptations may appear. Family dynamics may suffer; dependence on medications may increase as well as overutilization of medical services. This creates a complex health situation, which is often difficult for the patient and medical professionals to unravel. It is, however, understandable that many patients end up down this path.

While getting medical attention sooner than later for serious concerns or red flags is essential to faster healing, this *does not* eliminate the importance of self-care. Pain is the body's alarm system for *perceived* threats or current dysfunction; remembering this is vital. Symptoms should not be ignored, even if the medical field cannot explain why pain is present. **Preventing a physical and emotional downward spiral should be a primary consideration while tending to self-care.**

A common issue among all chronic pain sufferers is *fear*. Uncertainty about recovery plays a role, but fear, in this case, is more about avoiding physical activities that bring about or exacerbate chronic pain. Called *fear-avoidance*, it is an area of recognized importance in the medical field. Three types of fear-avoiders are typically described:[22]

***Misinformed* avoiders** believe pain indicates harm and that the spine is vulnerable. This belief is unfounded since the spine is carefully protected within the body. However, misinformed avoiders will go out of their way to feel safe, including limiting activity.

***Learned* avoiders** do not see pain as a problem, but they think pain should be avoided. To achieve this goal, learned avoiders limit all healthy activity, which can cause additional problems.

***Affective* avoiders** may place a distorted significance on pain and have concerns about conditions of the spine. Anxiety and depression are hallmarks of this avoider along with a significant reduction of all activities that might trigger pain. *Addressing anxiety and depression is crucial to improve perceived suffering.*

Yet, some pain sufferers may be none of the above, but could be labeled as "pain-endurers" or "fear-fighters." These strong-willed types overpower any fear of injury or pain with a more prevailing desire to maintain previous function *at all costs*. Yet, by not acknowledging or listening to the body, the pain persists and/or the body finds other ways to get the body to slow down and pay attention.[23]

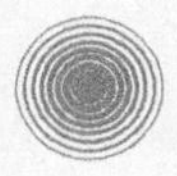

"Pain is the body's alarm system for *perceived* threats or current dysfunction."

There is some evidence to suggest that excessive levels of fear-avoidance behaviors, both in patients and in health professionals, have a negative impact on low back pain outcomes because the behaviors delay recovery and heighten disability.[24] In other words, by not educating patients and implementing unfounded physical restrictions, physicians may be fueling patient fears and inadvertently worsening their pain and function. **Education is important for all types of avoiders, but it is of utmost importance for those patients who believe experiencing pain is harmful.**[25]

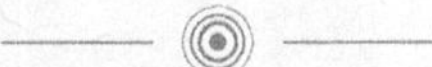

In this first section of the book, many aspects of pain and the human body reveal how fascinating yet perplexing pain can truly be. To add insult to injury, navigating through the medical system in search of answers can leave patients even more frustrated. The next section provides as complete a picture as possible of the capabilities and limitations of medicine today, especially in the field of chronic pain.

PART 2

THE MEDICAL SYSTEM

CHAPTER 6

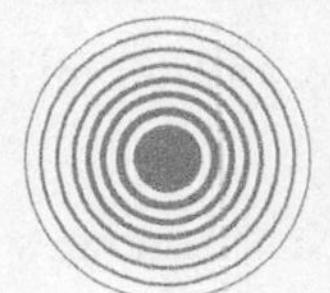

Today's Medical Business

Economic medicine that was previously meted out by the cupful has recently been dispensed by the barrel. These once unthinkable dosages will almost certainly bring on unwelcome after-effects. Their precise nature is anyone's guess, though one likely consequence is an onslaught of inflation.

—**Warren Buffett**

The field of medicine is a *business*. Hospitals, clinics, and medical practices all have expenses that must be paid in order to create profit. Patients are the consumers of the medical industry. If a self-employed physician does not have a cash-only practice, then the physician usually ends up signing contracts with insurance companies or other systems. The physician who agrees to insurance contracts is enabling a third party to make a profit on top of the actual costs of health services—sad, but true. It would appear the good news for physicians is that with so many patients mandated to have insurance, they have a larger pool of potential patients with which to fill their practices. However, the physician's *worth* is dictated by the medical insurance company—in other words, the insurance company will only agree to pay a percentage for each of the services rendered to patients. At first blush, medical insurance appears to be a good thing for patients. It allows patients to receive services that might otherwise be out of reach financially. However, just as this system helps, it also hinders. Insurance companies, not the direct physician, often dictate the care, the physician's value, and the treatments patients receive. This is inherently wrong, and the ill health of the U.S. population reflects this backward notion.

With traditional health insurance, any visit to a physician generates three costs. First, there is the cost that the patient pays, usually a *copay or coinsurance*. Second, there is the *billed cost*—the actual cost of the service. Third, there is the *actual amount paid to the physician* by the insurance provider. Many times that amount paid to the physician is only a percentage of the billed cost. For example, a physician may only be paid 15 percent of the amount billed to the insurance provider for a visit or treatment. In other words, a $100 visit would only net $15 from the insurance company. The physician's *billed cost* is not usually paid in full.

In order to be paid that $15, much work must be done in physicians' offices just to cover the cost of getting a patient's payment from an insurance company. Many times nearly half of the overhead business costs of medical practices are for the personnel cost needed to obtain payment from the patients' insurance companies. As an example, if consumers could purchase the Apple iPhone with insurance, Apple would have to spend almost half of its revenue just to obtain payment from insurance companies. The iPhone would need to cost significantly more if Apple wanted to continue making the same profit margin as before the insurance system started. There also probably would be a change in the employee culture and satisfaction with salaries at Apple if the workload and sales had to double to compensate for the lower profit margins. Realistically, Apple is too savvy to fall into this insurance scenario.

Here is another example. Suppose a change in the auto insurance industry mandated that all car maintenance and oil changes must be covered via insurance. Auto insurance payments would skyrocket as insurance companies scrambled to cover these new (and frequent) costs. An unfortunate twist in the system would mean that auto insurance policyholders would also bear the brunt of costs for car owners who don't maintain their vehicles well, requiring them to have bigger maintenance and service woes. Should everyone bear the burden of the excessive or avoidable use of the auto insurance's pool of financial resources? Society pays in the end. The less individuals take responsibility for controllable factors, then the more society bears the risk of the financial burden. There is only so much money to go around within a closed system, especially if the business entity expects some level of profit. The medical insurance world is no different.

Physicians *employed* by a hospital or business entity don't have it any easier with the current insurance reimbursement issues. In many cases, physicians must generate enough revenue to keep business investors happy and make a profit beyond the overhead costs. To accomplish the financial goals, physicians may run those practices like assembly lines. In other words, physicians may be heavily encouraged to perform a certain number of procedures per number of patients in order to meet the investors' revenue expectations. With physicians churning through patients, it is no wonder little time is spent emphasizing valuable life skills or education with patients.

It all comes back to poor reimbursement by insurance companies, which increases the need for higher patient volumes and services with higher financial return. This affects chronic pain patients because the quickest and most lucrative options—for physicians, CEOs, and medical industry middlemen—are injections, surgeries, and multiple brief office visits with little time to do anything but offer prescriptions. These approaches are typically a quick way to make the patient feel as if the pain complaint is being acknowledged and addressed, but each approach carries a host of problems that may result from its use.

On a side note, there is a growing desire from insurance or regulatory agencies to use "pay for performance" as a stipulation for payment to providers or hospitals. For example, if a diabetic's glycohemoglobin (HgA1c) lab value is not below a certain level, then the insurance provider may reimburse less for services rendered by the physician. Pay for performance is misdirected as it penalizes the physician with a smaller payment, even though the physician is not in full control of the situation. It does not account for *patient* performance. There are two sides of the coin here.

The reality is our society is continuing to deflect the patient's responsibility for optimizing health from within while physicians have no money incentive to emphasize the importance of self-care. **This passive approach to health with opioids, injections, and surgeries may put more money into the deep pockets of profiting businesses, but it is eroding the abilities of patients to enhance their own health.** This affects everyone's quality of life now and in the future.

Two additional flaws within the business of medicine include the system's elimination of the *artistic* component of medicine, which is not reimbursable and the need for *common sense*, which is not always supported by research. Similar to the complexity of pain, if fixing the medical system was simple, then it would be fixed already. Unfortunately, irrational methods have permeated most aspects of health care and left little financial incentive to spend time truly caring for patients or doing what makes sense. As the saying goes, "Common sense is not common practice."

In a larger context, common sense would suggest dealing with the *cause* of the health care crisis. Putting bandages on the inflation of health care only leads to more symptoms—in other words, further escalation of costs. Just like physicians with patients, society should focus on understanding and addressing causes, not just symptoms, of increased health care costs. Focusing on helping everyone "afford" medical care via mandated insurance makes it easier to ignore the causes of expensive health care. Much of the escalation of health care costs is related to overutilization of resources and excessive profit.

Profit is not evil per se; it allows businesses to continue to exist and to provide valuable services. Greed, however, is the unenviable quality embedded within this country's medical system. For instance, there is a lack of government regulation or control on hospitals, pharmaceuticals, medical device companies, or other medical system players to keep prices from running out of control.[26] In addition, patients and physicians do not know the actual cost of items or services at the time the medical services are rendered. This lack of transparency in an insurance-driven market enables an indiscriminate demand and burden on the medical system's resources, of which there is a finite supply.

Despite limited resources, government and politics are perpetuating the profits of the medical intermediaries by pulling more patients into the medical insurance system, as dictated now by U.S. law. This, in turn, continues the cycle of paying the exorbitant prices of all the uncontrolled medical players. Sadly, patients think they are getting a great deal when they get health insurance, but in reality there are many hidden profits being made off those insurance premiums. In addition, not every medical service or procedure is covered by insurance plans. One of the leading causes of personal bankruptcy is medical debt, *regardless of insurance status*. Having insurance will not protect the American public from prices that rise out of control. **Too much profit is being made at the expense of unsuspecting patients.**[27] It is unknown how long this can be sustained.

If patients are forced to have medical insurance, then the patient or the contributor (e.g., employer) is putting money in the third party's "bank" to use in alignment with the insurance plan's rules. There are monthly or yearly premium payments plus a deductible, which must be met by the patient before certain benefits kick in. Instead of a patient paying a physician directly for a service that is reasonably priced, an insurance company uses the pool of money to pay for a portion of the patient's expensive medical services *and its overhead* including the CEO salary, which can be from millions up to $30 million dollars![28]

Physicians in a standard clinical practice make pennies in comparison with many insurance CEOs. Yet despite CEOs lack of direct patient care, they are extracting a large amount of money from the potentially available funds for patients. This issue goes beyond CEOs of insurance companies—hospitals, medical device companies, and pharmaceutical companies are all trying to get a piece of the insurance system's money to fuel their own profits and enormous salaries.

It is not the same old supply and demand of old since the medical intermediaries have entered the game. The middlemen in the medical field have shifted the dynamics, and patients are unaware of all the decisions and negotiations that occur between insurance companies and the medical industry. **Because patients do not have immediate and obvious transparency with all the forces involved, they do not realize the cost to themselves and society when they make health care decisions.**

By agreeing to higher risk and more expensive treatments or procedures, patients are unwittingly contributing to the overutilization and higher costs of health care. What is best for profit-driven companies is not always necessary for the patient, especially if it has increased risk and limited benefit. Are some companies driven by what's right for the patient? Of course, those companies exist, but there is also no doubt that there are other businesses making ridiculous sums of money at the risk of patient health.

The medical industry works under a complicated and flawed business model fueled, in part, by the expansion of insurance coverage starting in the 1950s to cover more than just catastrophic events and by the lack of price controls throughout the industry. Patients have no idea what medical services and procedures truly cost, thus, disrupting the natural supply and demand economics between the physician and the patient—or "consumer" in the *business* of medicine. The once transparent system is clouding not just cost, but knowing who makes the rules nowadays. Fixing this broken system goes beyond the patient and physician. The political and governmental fabric is so deeply woven within the medical industry that it may take decades to change.

Unfortunately, non-medical personnel working within the medical industry, such as within an insurance company, do not wholly appreciate that medicine is not straightforward nor meant to be fragmented—yet, they are regulating patient care as if it is clear-cut. This leads to an algorithmic approach, which does not apply to or work for each individual. Humans are more complex than an automated and de-personalized algorithm. Personalized medicine is an art that advocates for the patient, not the pocket or convenience of the medical system. As long as more emphasis is placed on the pocket or convenience, then harm to the patient will occur more frequently than necessary.

Medical insurance can be a double-edged sword. You can use it to get services paid for which are *not necessary*. Yet, you can be *denied* coverage or payment for things that are important or *necessary* for your overall health and wellness. Denial of medical claims is all too common nowadays. **What is rational in the practice of *thoughtful* medicine is impractical for the system. It is a battle that patients and physicians fight every day in the United States.**

The flaws of today's medical system or *business* are deeply embedded within the American culture, requiring diligence, patience, and advocacy in order to actively pursue, navigate, and determine the optimal health care for pain.

CHAPTER 7

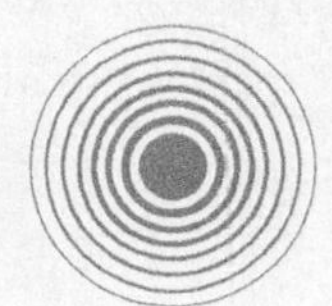

Different Approaches in Medicine

There are, in truth, no specialties in medicine, since to know fully many of the most important diseases a man must be familiar with their manifestations in many organs.

—**William Osler**, "Father of Modern Medicine"

It is intriguing how many different branches of medicine have come into being over the last 100 years. In an effort to improve the health of humans, society started to recognize that there must be better ways of doing things. Addressing trauma and infections were a big part of the advances of medicine; other issues have created challenges, including pain. If humans knew it all and one way worked, then there would be *little to no* desire or inclination to approach health in a different manner. It seems obvious, but the point is that humans are always seeking answers in various ways. Here are a few of the most commonly referenced approaches to medicine.

Mainstream Medicine (also referred to as Conventional or Western Medicine)

A system in which medical doctors or other healthcare professionals treat symptoms and diseases using drugs, radiation, or surgery.[29]

For low back pain complaints, mainstream medicine typically means a standard visit with a primary doctor for a brief history and physical, the ordering of a magnetic resonance image (MRI), and a surgeon or pain medicine referral.

Within mainstream medicine, there are two types of physicians in the United States:

Allopathic Medicine: Doctors of Medicine **(M.D.)** are commonly referred to as *allopathic* physicians by proponents of alternative medicine. M.D.s are physicians who use pharmacologically active agents or physical interventions to treat or suppress diseases or symptoms.[30] This is the most commonly encountered traditional physician in the United States. There are over 140 medical schools leading to the M.D. degree in North America, and there are more schools planned for the near future.

Osteopathic Medicine: Osteopathic physicians are Doctors of Osteopathy **(D.O.)** who are licensed to practice medicine and surgery in all 50 states and are recognized in over 40 other countries, including all Canadian provinces. There are currently more than 30 U.S. medical schools that lead to the D.O. degree—and more are coming.[31] Thus, the percentage of medical graduates who are D.O.s is smaller in number than M.D.s. Although M.D. material is covered in the D.O. curriculum, a distinct difference in *osteopathic* medical schools is the training in osteopathic manipulative medicine and the osteopathic philosophy, which includes these four major principles:[32]

1. The body is a unit; the person is a unit of body, mind, and spirit.
2. The body is capable of self-regulation, self-healing, and health maintenance.
3. Structure and function are reciprocally interrelated.

4. Rational treatment is based upon an understanding of the basic principles of body unity, self-regulation, and the interrelationship of structure and function.

Note, *osteopathy* in other parts of the world may refer to an "osteopath" who specializes solely in musculoskeletal or manual therapy work but is *not* a physician who can prescribe medication or perform surgery. To add to the confusion, some osteopaths (i.e., European) may refer to themselves as D.O.s, even if they are not physicians. It essentially depends on where the training was *received*; U.S.-trained osteopathic physicians are D.O.'s who *do* practice the full scope of medicine.

Complementary and Alternative Medicine

The term *complementary and alternative medicine* (CAM) is used extensively today, either separately or together. *Alternative* medicine usually refers to using a non-mainstream approach *in place of* conventional medicine. *Complementary* medicine usually refers to using a non-mainstream approach *together with* conventional medicine. Ironically, some *alternative* fields of medicine have become *complementary* as conventional medicine becomes more accepting of its use, such as acupuncture and massage.

Many patients describe their use of CAM out of a desire for a more holistic approach to their health. **Holistic care refers to the medical care of the whole person, including the mind, body, and soul, not just the symptom.** Regardless of where health care providers start in their education, some of them evolve through their practices to be more holistic than others do. Unfortunately, many patients living with chronic pain are frequently evaluated using a symptom-focused approach, a decidedly non-holistic view.

Integrative Medicine

The term *integrative medicine* has emerged recently and is defined as:

> *The practice of medicine that reaffirms the importance of the relationship between practitioner and patient, focuses on the whole person, is informed by*

evidence, and makes use of all appropriate therapeutic approaches, healthcare professionals and disciplines to achieve optimal health and healing.[33]

Both D.O.s and M.D.s can become board-certified in integrative medicine through the American Board of Physician Specialties. The emphasis in integrative medicine is on overall wellness and healing, whether it is using alternative, complementary, or mainstream practices. As in other specialties, there is variability among physicians within the practice of integrative medicine. It seems to be a practical approach if the best there is to offer from *all* realms of medicine is at the physician's disposal, but there will always be critics who question the existence or the need for "integrative" medicine. Yet, it is decidedly holistic, if practiced that way.

Regardless of how a certain school of medical thought is labeled, it is a disservice to not look at the patient with the broadest view possible. **A holistic approach makes sense from a general health perspective, but it makes even more sense when considering chronic pain, which is usually too complex to focus only on symptoms.** Some pain issues are straightforward as in a splinter. The removal of the splinter will typically take care of the sensory input associated with the perception of pain. Chronic pain is rarely that simple. Utilizing a holistic approach to chronic pain gives the physician other "tools" with which to assess, address, and assist a patient, including exploring mind, body, and lifestyle issues that may be contributing to chronic pain.

Through common sense, experience, and continuing research, the medical field can develop better ideas of how to address pain in a more *holistic* manner to minimize harm. Many components of the osteopathic philosophy are hidden within complementary, alternative, holistic, and integrative philosophies. In truth, the philosophies taught during initial medical training, however, do not always define the physician in practice—as in the M.D. who practices holistically and the D.O. who practices conventionally, not holistically. **The physician's title does not necessarily reveal the thought process or philosophy that a physician develops after years of clinical experience and study.**

Further, if a physician claims to be "holistic," it is still acceptable to get a second opinion if there are no conservative options discussed or offered for *non-urgent* issues. Not every physician is a good fit, but it is also important for patients to engage in effective communication with the physician. When suffering from chronic pain, it is important to identify the best health professional and treatment options for the individual, not simply do what friends/neighbors/boss did when they had pain issues.

Whether because of blind faith in their physician's opinion or a desperate decision made in the hopes of pain relief, patients are agreeing to take on more risk with procedures, especially when the methods are commonplace or socially acceptable. Patients are only familiar with what they have seen, heard, or been taught. Currently, society seems to get more "education" from their inner circle of friends or outside business marketing than from physicians. To compound the problem, society and physicians are not always instructing patients on better alternatives. The physicians may be well-intentioned, but they only do what they have been taught or learned along the way. These physicians may believe they are being conservative by suggesting injections or medications versus surgery, but risky drugs and interventions are offered too quickly and may not address the *cause* of the pain problem. If physicians are not taught to be holistic and evaluate other possibilities, then it is more likely that the cause or contributor to a patient's pain will be missed.

Conversely, holistic physicians regularly recommend a conservative treatment first. Not only may the patient be unimpressed by a lack of "technology," but this less-invasive approach can have the unintended consequence of disappointing the patient if the therapy/treatment/procedure is ineffectual. The patient may then believe if one type of conservative therapy does not work, then nothing will—causing the patient to throw in the towel too soon. This is where good communication between patient and physician can make a difference. Educating the patient on the treatment plan trajectory gives the holistic physician a much better chance of helping the patient become as pain-free as possible. The physician also enables the patient to be a partner in treatment decisions. Success is more likely when patients are invested in their health and actively involved in the care of their bodies.

Sometimes it takes time in the medical field to realize that what physicians are doing or not doing can be harmful to their patients. There are plenty of illustrations in this country's past to recognize that brainwashing or indoctrinating the public with ideas or options that appeal to emotion or immediate gratification can be far from appropriate or ethically sound. For instance, in the middle part of the 20th century, physicians were convinced that smoking cigarettes was a healthy pastime. It is unlikely that a physician would recommend a patient take up smoking today. Yet, there does seem to be a fascination, glamorization even, of taking a pill, having surgery, or eating unhealthy foods. **Appealing to emotions, immediate gratification, and passivity of the American public is enabling a sicker society.** The politics and profits that fuel that emphasis are not easy to fight. The responsibility falls on the physician to be wary of negative influences on the practice of medicine, but it is equally important for patients to be invested in their own health.

If mainstream medicine in the U.S. was truly educating physicians on the value of nutrition, fitness, psychological, and biomechanical health, there would not be so many unhealthy, unfit, chronically fatigued, and unhappy physicians, many of whom also suffer with chronic pain. While it is true that working within the health care system is stressful or "painful," patients model what they see and hear. If physicians are not emphasizing or demonstrating the very real value of healthy living, then why would anyone expect patients to understand its importance? This is not a slam on my colleagues or me; however, unless physicians become, as Gandhi put it, "…the change you wish to see in the world," health care's focus on symptoms versus the whole person will not evolve.

The segmenting of medicine into the health care labels of alternative, complementary, conventional, or any specific approach that chooses one vantage point at the exclusion of others does not serve patients well. By collaborating and being open to exploring areas of medicine that are not well understood, such as pain, then medicine can become less fragmented and *whole* again. Until then, **it is up to patients and physicians to educate themselves about the different approaches available throughout medicine to create a more logical and holistic approach to optimal health.**

CHAPTER 8

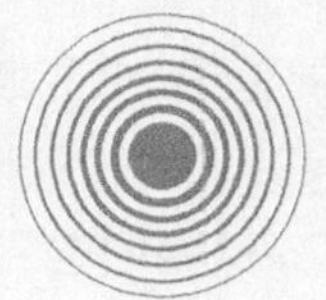

The Opioid Fiasco

Currently available treatments have limited effectiveness for most people with severe chronic pain.

—**Institute of Medicine**, *Relieving Pain in America: A Blueprint for Transforming Prevention, Care, Education, and Research*

When a patient presents with chronic, often debilitating pain, the conventional physician faces a few choices after the examination and symptoms discussion. The question of whether the physician can "make the pain go away" may not have an easy answer, especially if the cause of the pain remains unknown. Whether the physician is big hearted, seeking to move on to the next patient or both, the prescription pad will likely appear, or a recommendation to a surgeon will be the result of the appointment. In fact, the most common outcomes for chronic pain patients are opioids, injections, and surgery.

While there is a time and a place for these treatments, all too often, their use is substantiated especially when patients are desperate for help or if it is believed those are the only options. These "solutions" rarely get to the heart of the matter. In fact, if medical professionals were doing such a great job of understanding or managing pain in the United States, there would not be a *Paindemic* on our hands.

Physicians could and should do a better job for patients by conducting further research, educating patients on alternatives, and developing strategies to treat the cause of health issues, not simply suppressing symptoms. Patients rely on physicians to provide them with current, relevant information. If patients are not exposed to other care options, they don't even have the opportunity to consider alternatives. I see this happen all too often. Physicians usually are not purposely misleading patients; rather, they may not *believe* in alternative therapies or they do not provide those services. In this scenario, the physician is making decisions for the patient, at least with regard to the information provided, eliminating the chance for patients to make fully informed choices about their care.

Based on how the information is presented, the patient may believe and trust the "diagnosis" and recommended treatment from the *first* physician consulted. However, **if there are no red flags and the first recommendation involves opioids or invasive procedures, I would suggest another opinion.** Patients should consider the types of providers they are seeing, and what each has to offer. Surgeons do surgery; pain medicine physicians typically offer pain medications or interventions. Some physicians are more conservative in their approach than others are. Some physicians have more experience and appreciate the limitations of their own interventions. **What patients choose to do in response to their pain can determine the quality of life now...and later.**

Continuous opioid use should never be a *first-line* option in chronic, non-cancer pain.[34,35] Physicians who emphasize highly advertised and riskier treatments bypass the importance of lower-risk options for chronic pain. The concept of "just take a pill and ease the pain" increases and encourages long-term passivity in patients. Physicians who ascribe to this method of doctoring do not give patients a chance to prove to themselves that they can improve their lives with better education, direction, and effort. This concept is similar to people who constantly eat sugar-laden, processed foods and do not feel that they can be satisfied by healthy foods such as fruits and vegetables. Mentally, there is already an exposure, a perceived benefit, and a predilection for a more seductive or powerful alternative, even if it is not in the person's best interest.

Powerful drugs, such as opioids, can only be prescribed predominantly by physicians. Therefore, many people use more convenient and less expensive over-the-counter pain relievers, such as acetaminophen and nonsteroidal anti-inflammatory drugs.

Acetaminophen

Most people in the U.S. and Japan are familiar with *acetaminophen* (e.g., Tylenol). The same drug, in the United Kingdom or Australia, is called *paracetamol.* Acetaminophen can be helpful in masking pain temporarily. It has weak anti-inflammatory properties, however, but can be useful for different types of pain. Many times, it is combined with stronger medications in the same pill. How acetaminophen works in the body is only partly understood, although research is ongoing. Typically, maximum daily dosage recommendations are 4000 milligrams per day, but this amount can vary. This is especially true if other medical issues are present such as liver disease. When a healthy person takes acetaminophen as directed, problems are rare. However, allergic reactions, liver damage (especially when used with alcohol), or overdoses can occur. Intentional or unintentional overdoses can lead to death within three to five days if emergency treatment is not effective. If the person survives, but the liver damage is severe, then a liver transplant would be necessary.

Nonsteroidal Anti-Inflammatory Drugs (NSAIDs)

Nonsteroidal anti-inflammatory drugs (NSAIDs) such as aspirin, ibuprofen, and naproxen can be quite effective at reducing pain through strong anti-inflammatory effects; however, these drugs are not without their risks. The type of NSAID and its dosing impact those risks differently. Gastrointestinal problems including ulcerations of the stomach lining and bleeding are well documented and can be life-threatening, especially if taking blood thinners or if advanced in age. For those who are more susceptible, kidney problems or kidney failure can arise due to changes in kidney blood flow. Elderly patients, who typically have lost some of their normal kidney function, can develop acute kidney failure within a week if they are susceptible to NSAIDs. Heart problems have also been reported with certain forms of NSAIDs. Some people can end up with salt retention, swelling, confusion, or dizziness. In pregnant women, a risk of miscarriage or premature birth is possible if NSAIDs are taken during the last trimester.

What is rarely discussed is the possibility that NSAIDs can be counterproductive for wound healing. Some inflammation is essential for healing, and areas that get very little blood supply such as tendons and ligaments may not receive an adequate inflammatory response to heal appropriately if taking NSAIDs.[36]

Adjuvant Medications

If over-the-counter pain medications are not working, physicians may prescribe *adjuvant medications*, which are not pain medicines per se but may be helpful in modifying the signals or experience of pain. Some of those include antidepressants, muscle relaxants, anti-seizure, anti-anxiety, or other medications, usually in the form of a pill, cream, or patch. All of these are targeted at modifying the nervous system's interpretation of pain, which requires a trial period to assess the medication's effectiveness with the patient's unique body response.

Opioids

When moderate to severe pain has not resolved, and the over-the-counter medications or adjuvant medications have not helped, physicians often turn to a plethora of opioids—the "big guns" in the pain reliever world. They are *opium-like compounds that affect one or more of at least three different receptors in the body.*

Opioids can be effective, but they come with an array of potential side effects such as mild to severe constipation, which slows down a critical bodily function. Chronic dry mouth can occur, leading to tooth decay.[37] Sex hormones and the immune system can be adversely affected as well.[38] Over time, a tolerance to the opioid's pain-relieving effects can develop, requiring higher doses for the same relief. On the flip side, a phenomenon called *opioid-induced hyperalgesia* can occur, whereby more pain medication actually *makes the pain worse*—seems counterintuitive but it can happen.[39] Fortunately, all of these side effects usually get better when the patient weans down or off the medication.

It has been discovered, however, that one aspect of continuous opioid treatment does not resolve even after the patient discontinues its use. A study evaluated patients who took *morphine for one month* and patients who did *not* take morphine for chronic low back pain. Researchers used MRI scans to evaluate the test subjects' brains before use, at one month of use, and at approximately four months after discontinuing the opioids.

After only one month, the brains of the opioid users clearly showed *neuroplastic* changes. The MRIs revealed multiple areas of the brain that *increased* in volume. However, the *right amygdala lost volume*. This finding was concerning because the *amygdala* is involved in drug-induced behaviors, drug craving, behavior reinforcement, and withdrawal. The higher the morphine dose, the more brain volume the subject lost in the amygdala. More troubling, many areas of the brain with opioid receptors *increased* in size after one month but *did not decrease* in size four months after discontinuing the opioids. Although it is being debated as to what the changes in brain size really mean, **there is evidence that opioids affect the size of brain matter while they are being used, but, once discontinued, the brain does NOT return to its original appearance for at least four months after discontinuing them.** Another brain area affected by opioids is the *hypothalamus*, which is responsible for releasing substances that control attention and wakefulness. Two common issues for people taking opioids are, not surprisingly, lethargy and inattention.[40]

Amid the opioid haze, *sedation and respiratory depression* can occur at different doses. If the dose is too high, it is possible to lose the natural drive to breathe. In addition, the longer acting the opioids are, the higher the risk goes. In fact, the risk of unintentional overdose injury or death is *twice* as high when given long-acting opioids versus short-acting opioids.[41] It is no wonder that the occurrence of opioid overdose deaths in the U.S. has skyrocketed over the last 20 years since opioids have been given more freely for non-cancer pain. This increased use is a bit shocking. Although Americans only comprise about five percent of the world's population, they use 80 percent of the world's opioid supply. Specifically,

Americans have consumed up to 99 percent of the world supply of hydrocodone, a derivative of codeine.[42,43]

This overuse of hydrocodone prompted a change in the way physicians prescribe or refill this powerful drug in October 2014. According to the Drug Enforcement Agency (DEA), a physician's office can no longer call in a prescription for a hydrocodone product (e.g., Norco, hydrocodone/acetaminophen). Any product containing hydrocodone was reclassified from a Schedule 3 to a Schedule 2 drug. This means a written prescription must be given to the patient to *hand-deliver* to the pharmacy—no more phone call refills. There are more rules being implemented to reduce access and increase opioid monitoring. This is one way to reduce opioid over-prescribing and subsequent over-use, but it makes getting these drugs more difficult for the *few* people who truly need them. In addition, for those who are dependent on the medications, do not have a prescription, and desperate for a replacement, many are turning to less-expensive heroin on the streets.[44]

In the past, many physicians used opioids only for cancer pain. This changed in the 1990s around the same time a New York physician, Dr. Russell Portenoy, argued that opioids could be used safely for *non-cancer* pain as well.[45,46] He was not the only proponent—other medical professionals and certain pharmaceutical companies such as Purdue Pharma were promoting the safety of opioids.[47,48] This misguided belief hinged on the fact that less than one percent of patients using opioids became addicted, and, at the time, it was extremely rare for a patient to overdose. This theory was not based on substantial evidence and was not monitored over a long period. Dr. Portenoy also campaigned as the president of the American Pain Society to make pain the "fifth vital sign" to establish the scoring protocol patients use to rate their pain from zero to 10, with 10 being the worst. The patient pain rating could then be used as part of the decision as to which pain medication to prescribe. With these changes, suddenly misguided physicians had a much larger selection of pain medications from which to choose and felt obligated to treat the pain "score." Yet with more opioids in the hands of patients, an eye-opening epidemic was emerging.

According to the Centers for Disease Control (CDC), **fatal opioid-related drug overdoses more than quadrupled between 1999 through**

2010. In 1999, 4,030 lost their lives to opioid-related overdoses; in 2010, that number was 16,651.[49] Unfortunately, many of these overdoses were the result of *mixing* alcohol or *benzodiazepines* (e.g., Xanax) with an opioid. Perhaps these deaths could have been prevented if the patient had not been taking an opioid, or if the patient understood the danger of mixing alcohol and other powerful drugs. Unfortunately, not all lives lost were "prescribed" opioids; diverted medications end up in the hands of family, friends, children, or strangers purchasing them for medical or non-medical reasons on the street. With the information available today, it is hoped that physicians carefully weigh the pros and cons of opioid use before prescribing them, especially in combination with other sedating medications.[50] There is **still insufficient evidence to understand how effective long-term opioids can be for improving chronic, non-cancer pain and function**. Despite this reality, 259 million painkiller prescriptions were prescribed in 2012 alone and approximately 46 people died *every day* from opioid-related overdoses.[51]

With opioid over-prescribing and subsequent overuse come interesting overdose reforms such as those being championed in multiple states with support from the American Society of Addiction Medicine. These reforms would allow emergency first-responders *and non-medical* individuals, such as family and friends, to administer a reversal agent, *naloxone*, to the suspected overdosing patient.[52,53] Naloxone is an *opioid antagonist* that stops an overdose, if given in time. It is effective, inexpensive, fast acting, and easy to administer into the nose or inject into the muscle of the overdosing patient. It is most effective before severe respiratory depression or respiratory arrest occurs. It is sad to me that we need reforms like this to undo a problem that was perpetuated by physicians prescribing too many opioids.

Has Opioid Use Really Gone Too Far?

Dr. Portenoy reflected on the opioid over-prescribing in a 2012 interview with the *Wall Street Journal*. He admitted it was "quite scary" that he may have contributed to the soaring rates of addiction and overdose deaths. He stated, "Clearly, if I had an inkling of what I know now then, I wouldn't have spoken in the way that I spoke. It was clearly the wrong thing to do."[54,55] Many physicians have realized this fact for themselves.

One of the most challenging and heartbreaking aspects of opioid over-prescribing in the last two decades is that many patients *started* on opioids *early*. They may have received them from a primary care physician, emergency medicine physician, pain medicine physician, or a surgeon. By the time they are sent to a pain medicine specialist, they may have been on opioids for a while and likely on other sedatives, such as a benzodiazepine (e.g., Xanax or Ativan). Combining opioids with benzodiazepines for long-term treatment of chronic, non-cancer pain is not recommended and tends to be associated with higher risk patients with more mental health conditions and higher rates of using emergency health care.[56,57] Trying to wean medications from those patients convinced that drugs are the only option, is extraordinarily difficult.

Unlike managing a caffeine withdrawal, which can result in severe headaches, opioid withdrawal can be worse. Removing opioids such as hydrocodone or oxycodone can leave the patient miserable with sweating, heightened anxiety, muscle aches, yawning, a runny nose, abdominal cramping, vomiting, or the inability to sleep. Even newborns born to opioid-dependent mothers have it rough if withdrawal symptoms arise after birth.[58] Withdrawal from opioids is not typically life-threatening, but the central nervous system does take a while to re-acclimate to life without the drugs. On the other hand, stopping or weaning too quickly off long-term *benzodiazepines* such as Xanax could be life-threatening due to seizures or mental instability along with a whole host of other unpleasant withdrawal effects.

Physicians face a difficult situation. With a poor understanding of pain within the medical field and limited effective tools in their toolbox, physicians were told to prescribe opioids if they choose, without worries of addiction. However, some patients can become addicted despite taking those medications as prescribed. The opioid fiasco with unnecessary deaths has pushed the pendulum in the other direction. Many regulatory agencies are starting to penalize and criminalize physicians for doing what they have been taught to do; yet, there is little education given to physicians for other alternatives. Physicians are recognizing they must create a regimented and depersonalized approach for regulating their patients *who begin or remain on opioids* via medication contracts, pharmacy limitations, and random urine drug screens. This approach can make patients feel judged for wanting their pain medications. Worst of all, trying to convince patients they do not need to stay on opioids for their chronic, non-cancer pain without clear alternatives is worse than taking candy from a child.

Whether addicted or not, discontinuing *long-term* opioid use can be difficult when the body is accustomed to the drug leading to uncomfortable withdrawal symptoms. Addiction medicine specialists can assist patients with weaning off opioids, especially those who are truly addicted and struggling with cravings unrelated to withdrawal.[59] These specialists are not always easily available, and it is another specialist that must be added to the laundry list of other medical professionals in that patient's life. The medical community has created problems for patients by indiscriminately prescribing unnecessary opioids, and now this same community expects patients to undo the consequences through yet another subspecialty. Further, while physicians encourage opioid weaning, patients are told to accept the pain without other explanations as to the cause of or solution to their chronic pain. That is a bitter pill for patients to swallow.

Opioids work by dampening the pain signals in the brain. Instead of the pain yelling, its volume is turned down or silenced. It is true that many people do well with careful use of narcotics, but they come at a price, literally and figuratively. For patients with a terminal illness who simply need comfort care, opioids may be worth the side effects. For people who have a non-cancer situation with a desire to get back into life and its activities, blunting or putting a bandage on the pain does nothing to determine the pain's cause. By not treating the cause early, then the true problem could progress and grow more complex, leading to decreased overall function. Treating patients in this way gives them a "double whammy." In other words, their bodies develop a tolerance to the opioids, and the original problem is not addressed. The result is a worsening pain problem along with increased dependence or tolerance to opioids.

Unfortunately, quieting the pain with opioids or procedures is the status quo for most traditional pain medicine practices. It is not uncommon for pain patients to be using more than 80-120 milligrams of morphine or its equivalent per day. If that medicine is being used for fibromyalgia, headaches, or chronic low back pain, then the risks likely outweigh the benefit.[60] A short course of opioids may help facilitate activity and motion, but the quality of life should improve with increased activity; otherwise, there is no reason to use opioids long-term.

Beyond the multiple health risks of taking medications, the financial cost of opioid use can be staggering. For example, the powerful opioid, oxycodone, taken twice a day could cost upwards of $200 per month (60 pills). Assuming that the patient was not on any other pain medications, the cost would be $2,400 per year *to just cover up the signal of their pain while incurring risks and never dealing with the actual cause of their pain.* Similarly, if a patient takes eight Norco (i.e., hydrocodone plus acetaminophen) pills each day, the cost could be almost $600 per month.[61] That could equate to $7,200 per year! These cost figures do not include other expenses, such as urine drug screening, frequent office visits, and other possible complications that may arise from opioid use.

Opioid "solutions" are fraught with all of the above concerns along with the dilemma of dependency on perpetual, repeated doses for relief; thus, necessitating more and more visits to the doctor for prescriptions. The risks and benefits of opioids should be heavily weighed against the goals of optimal health and good function. **All things considered, the "opioid fiasco" is a reminder that using opioids can be a slippery slope—so, proceed with caution!**

CHAPTER 9

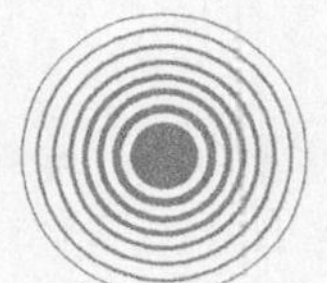

Conventional Pain Medicine Procedures

I suppose it is tempting, if the only tool you have is a hammer, to treat everything as if it were a nail.

—**Abraham Maslow**, *Toward a Psychology of Being*

Beyond opioid use, other conventional approaches that can assist with *symptom management* include a variety of interventional techniques ranging from trigger point injections to implantable pain pumps. This chapter will highlight some of the most common interventions used in traditional pain medicine clinics, and most of them will expose the patient to brief radiation at each encounter. Since approaches can vary and evolve over time, additional information can be found online, in books, or ultimately from a pain physician regarding how these procedures are performed.

Before any invasive approach is undertaken, the physician should provide a thorough description of what to expect, the risks, and the benefits of such a procedure. A second opinion, or even a third, is warranted before jumping into either opioids or procedures described in this chapter. Full disclosure empowers patients. Physicians who refuse or are unable to speak frankly about treatments and procedures should be avoided. Furthermore, before pursuing invasive procedures, the prudent physician should insist on various *noninvasive* therapies, even though these are not usually as profitable. The ultimate goal would be to facilitate increased range of motion, improve daily function, or enhance participation in physical or manual therapy.

Most of the brief injection procedures *do not require* sedation, especially heavy sedation. Many physicians, however, are offering full sedation for patients who demand it. Yet most procedures are only a few minutes long, and patients receiving repeated sedation get accustomed to not learning skills to handle "discomfort." Again, passivity when unnecessary is not helpful for patients in the long run. Heavy (unconscious) sedation comes with a greater risk, especially if the procedure involves the spine. This is because patients undergoing a spine treatment are typically face down on the table, which makes managing their breathing during heavy sedation more challenging. It is not uncommon for patients to have significant respiratory depression or obstruction, especially if they have obstructive sleep apnea. On occasion, patients can regurgitate or aspirate excess acid or stomach contents while unconscious—a primary reason for asking patients not to eat for approximately eight hours before sedation. Asking the pain physician who *handles the airway* (i.e., helps with breathing) in the event of an emergency during sedation is wise.

Unfortunately, many medical practice *business* models do not offer the *ideal* situation for patient safety if they do not have medical professionals trained in managing the airway. Instead, speed in the medical field is termed "efficiency," and irrational efforts to decrease overhead expenses seems to be the status quo in an insurance-driven business. Any infringement by non-medical businesspeople to demand excessive volume or accept less qualified personnel in medical practice settings is leading to more stressful and dangerous situations for patients, whether either party realizes it or not. This is, in part, why no sedation or the light (conscious) sedation route is safer. Some pain patients may present challenges for physicians without heavy sedation, but those are the exceptions.

Diagnostic Injections/Blocks

Most injections or blocks are used to *diagnose* the nerve sending unpleasant stimuli from the nerve cell receptor (nociceptor) to the brain; hence, *diagnostic* blocks or injections. Local anesthetic or numbing medicine is used to block the nerve from sending the receptor's pain stimuli up to the spinal cord and brain. Depending upon the *type* of local anesthetic chosen, pain relief typically lasts anywhere from one to eight hours. The caveat is that in some cases pain relief can last beyond the duration of the local anesthetic, whether it is for days, weeks, months, or longer. It is not completely understood who will have this type of response, or exactly how it occurs, but perhaps the nerve disruption or the relaxation of the associated connective tissue or musculature may have been enough for the body to discontinue its perception of pain.

If the pain was eliminated or decreased significantly at least for the duration of the local anesthetic injection and then subsequently returns, then a different procedure to *destroy* the nerve may be an option for longer pain relief. A variety of techniques can be used to accomplish nerve destruction: *radiofrequency ablation* (electrical/heat), *chemoablation* (chemical), or *cryoablation* (cold). All can prolong pain relief *until the nerve heals or grows back.*

The following are examples of diagnostic blocks:

Medial branch blocks are targeted primarily for suspected facet (or *zygapophyseal*) joint pain in the spine while using fluoroscopy or live X-ray guidance. (see Figure 2) The medial branch nerves are *not* visible under X-ray, but the physician knows where the nerves *usually* live in most people. A small amount of local anesthetic is injected at that location, and a review of the patient's initial response is made within 30 minutes after the injection or later. Under certain circumstances, the facet joints can be targeted directly by placing the needle inside the joint capsule. A small amount of steroid may be used with facet joint injections.

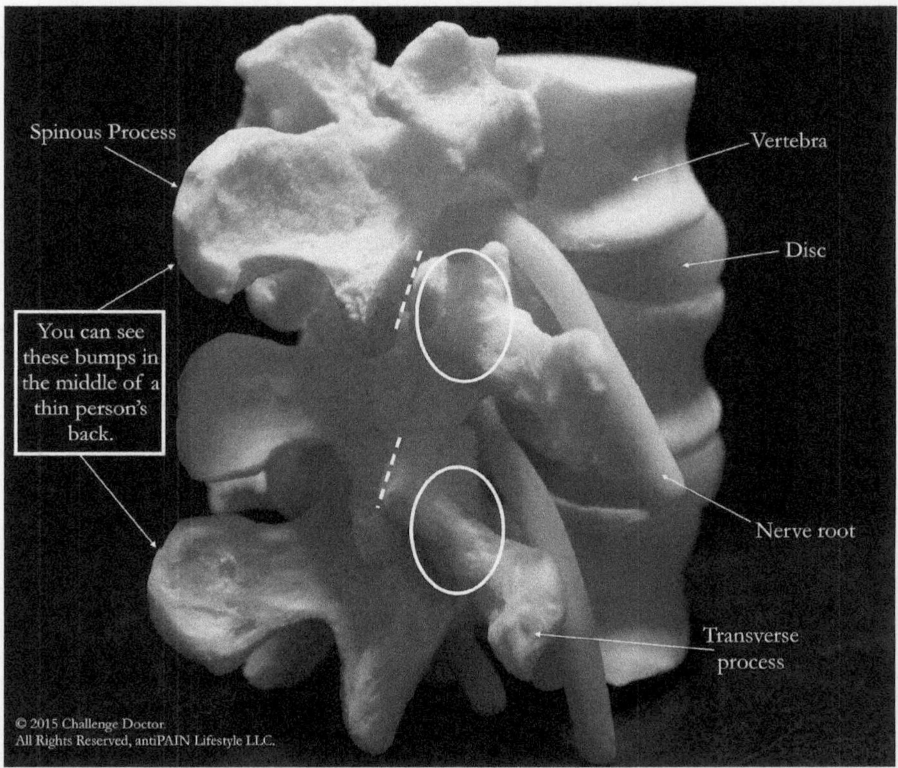

Figure 2: Medial Branch Block (MBB). This is a section of a spine model. The area that is targeted in a MBB is in the vicinity of the circled areas. Fluoroscopy or live X-ray does *not* show the actual medial branch nerves, but the area where they tend to live is targeted. A thin needle is guided to that area, and contrast is injected to verify that the needle is not obviously in a blood vessel or other area. If no concerns, then the numbing medicine is injected. Medial branch nerves do not *only* supply the facet joint [depicted by dashed lines], but also nearby muscles and connective tissues.

Selective nerve blocks can be used throughout the body for a variety of small, peripheral nerves. For instance, the *lateral femoral cutaneous nerve*, which is located in the upper outer portion of the thigh, can be injected with local anesthetic to see if the associated pain is relieved.

Discograms are used to decipher if and which disc is causing the pain. A needle is inserted into the suspected intervertebral disc in addition to one or two other discs. Contrast may be injected into each of those discs in an attempt to reproduce the original pain complaint. If the suspected disc is the only one causing pain during the procedure, then that disc is targeted for treatment, possibly surgery. However, there is some evidence to suggest that this procedure, which *invasively targets the disc*, accelerates degenerative disc disease because the disc's original integrity has been violated.[62] In addition, injecting into discs that are not typically painful could still cause pain.[63] For these and other reasons, this procedure is not as common as others are nowadays.

Sympathetic Nerve Blocks can be used for conditions such as complex regional pain syndrome (CRPS), which is a dysfunction of the *sympathetic nervous system* (SNS). The SNS is part of your "fight or flight" system. When escaping a lion or other threat, the body is on high alert with a variety of chemical changes occurring that enhance the ability to run away. With CRPS, the body generates an *excessive* fight or flight response, which *persists* in one extremity or area, although it can expand to other areas. CRPS can be expressed by a constellation of symptoms such as prolonged or excessive pain, variable skin color changes, temperature changes, and/or swelling to the affected area. If the symptoms are predominantly in the *arm*, then a *stellate ganglion block* may be performed. A *ganglion* is a cluster of nerve cell bodies and, in this case, is part of the sympathetic nervous system. This block is performed with the assistance of ultrasound and/or fluoroscopy to target an area adjacent to the level of the spine at approximately the sixth cervical vertebra (although approaches can vary). With important nearby structures, there is increased potential for complications, especially if the physician is not experienced. In the event pain symptoms are in the *legs*, then a *lumbar sympathetic ganglion* can be targeted. A lumbar sympathetic nerve block is performed for leg pain related to CRPS using fluoroscopy to target and inject medication at the level of the second lumbar vertebra (aka L2).

Nerve Destruction or Ablation Methods

Some of the diagnostic blocks above are done once or twice to determine if the patient experiences enough relief from the injected local anesthetic, at least for the lifespan of the numbing medicine. If the relief was adequate for that short period of time but the pain returned, then injuring or damaging the nerves is usually the next step to get longer relief. Again, *radiofrequency ablation* (electrical/heat), *chemoablation* (chemical), and *cryoablation* (cold) are some of the ways that this can be accomplished. If destroyed successfully, the nerve is no longer capable of sending the stimuli to the spinal cord or brain to be interpreted as pain. Sometimes sedation is used for radiofrequency procedures, as they can be too uncomfortable for some patients if not enough local anesthetic is used.

Destruction of the nerves, as in radiofrequency ablation of the medial branches, can lead to unintended consequences. The medial branch nerves supply not only the facet joints, but also other areas nearby such as some of the back muscles, overlying connective tissue, and skin. Because the nerve is destroyed, the muscles can atrophy or become weak. Without the nerve firing to that muscle for months or until the nerve grows back, there is no input to maintain muscle strength or tone. How long it takes to recover that strength, to what extent it can be recovered, and whether there are any long-term consequences to the patient's body and function are still yet to be understood.[64]

Trigger Point Injections

Trigger point injections are also used to diagnose and treat chronic pain. They are typically injected into the most tender spots of the muscle to relax it or the associated connective tissue and potentially relieve the pain for the duration of the local anesthetic or longer. These are typically done as needed with local anesthetic only and no steroid. At times, *botulinum toxin* (e.g., Botox) may be used in hopes of longer relief but there can be risks, such as swallowing or speech problems when using too much in the neck area. There is some debate about the reason for the benefits of this technique and who is most likely to benefit from it. Yet, many people seem to find great relief from trigger point injections despite challenges in obtaining solid research to explain the nature of "trigger points."[65,66]

Sacroiliac Joint Injections

Sacroiliac joint (aka SI joint) injections address suspected sacroiliac joint pain, which is a frequent area of low back pain. (see Figure 3) The joint injection can help with diagnosis but also can be therapeutic, such as with the smaller *facet* joints mentioned earlier. The needle enters the large joint, or as close as possible, to place local anesthetic and/or steroid medication; however, the benefits of the steroid versus just local anesthetic are variable. If there is difficulty with getting into the joint space, then there are alternative ways similar to *medial branch block injections* to help with sacroiliac joint pain. If there is pain relief, it does not mean that the body's function or movement has improved; however, it may enable better performance in daily activities or facilitate therapy leading to less pain. In addition, this does *not* mean that SI joint pain is due to a deficiency of local anesthetic requiring frequent injections. The pain can be due to a local inflammatory joint problem, but most of the time it could be due to the area's vulnerability to strains from poor or non-neutral body mechanics, which can be hard to prove in studies.[67,68,69,70,71,72,73,74]

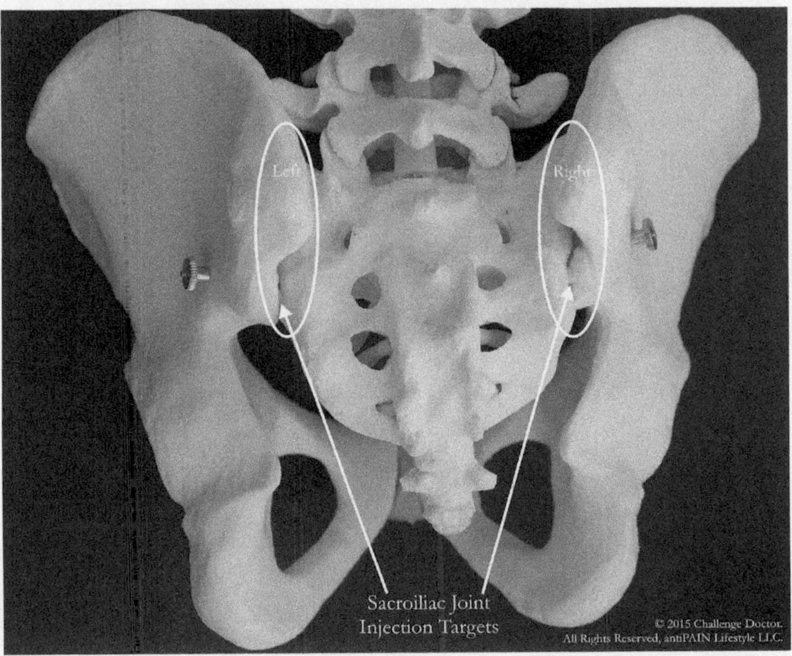

Figure 3: When injecting into the sacroiliac joint (aka SI joint), it is usually easier to approach this complex joint from the lower portion, as depicted by the arrows.

Diagnostic Spinal Block

On rare occasion, a spinal block, which is used frequently for scheduled cesarean sections, can be used to decipher if lower body pain is due to information from the body or strictly from the brain. A small amount of local anesthetic is injected into the lower spinal sac to create a complete block of sensation and motion of the lower body from around the waist level down to the feet. (see Figure 4) For instance, if someone has pain at the anus despite having a full spinal block in place, then it is assumed the patient has *central pain. Central pain* refers to pain originating from the central nervous system (e.g., brain). In other words, if there is still anal pain but the numbing medicine prevents signals from travelling

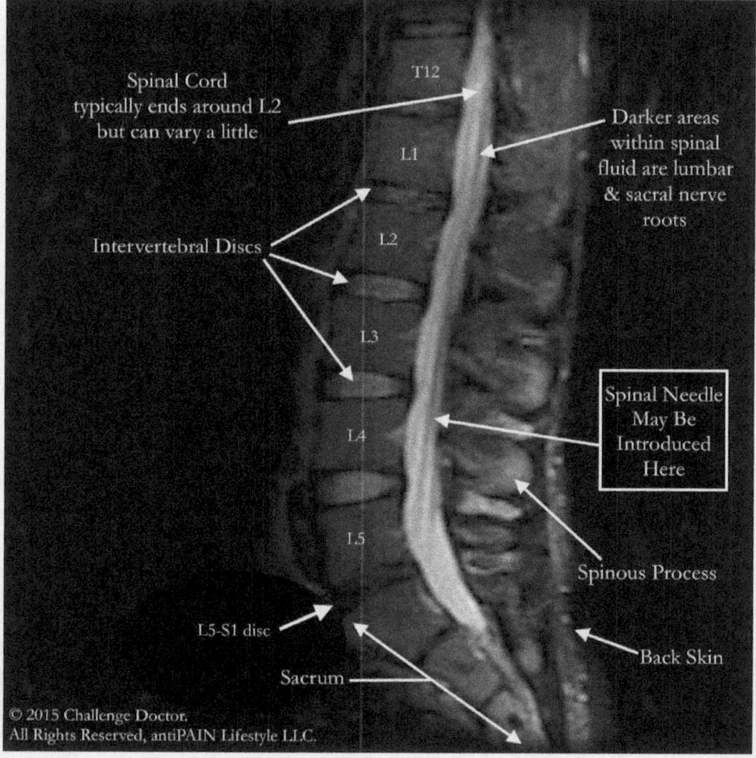

Figure 4: A spinal is performed while the patient is sitting, face down, or lying on one side. A spinal needle is used to place numbing medicine *within the spinal sac below the spinal cord*, where the lowest nerve roots are floating within the spinal fluid.

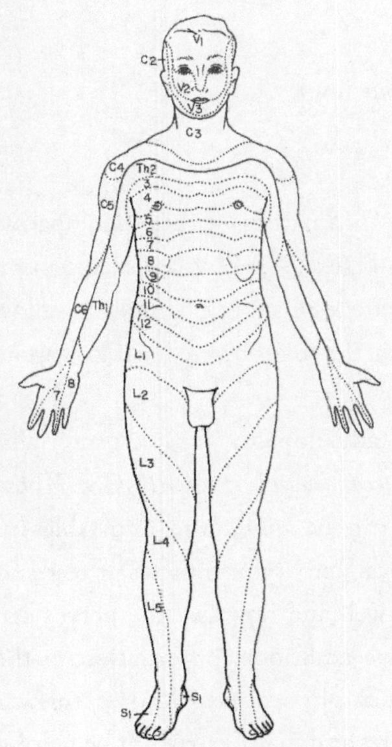

Figure 5: Although everywhere, the dermatomes on the front of the body are illustrated here. Each dermatome takes a path from the spine around to the front of the body. Pain or numbness related to nerve root problems typically follow one of the dermatome pathways seen here. Yet, not everyone fits this estimated mapping precisely. *Permission to use from Wolters Kluwer Health:* Bonica's *The Management of Pain*, 2nd ed., ed. John J. Bonica et al. (Philadelphia: Lea and Febiger, 1990): 139.

from the anus to the brain, then the pain is truly maintained in the brain. It is implied that treating the pain at the site where the patient senses the pain, such as the anus, would not do any good. In that case, the patient would be treated with medication or other therapies to address the central nervous system, not the anus. Cutting out the anus would do no good either.

Epidural Steroid Injections

Unsurprisingly, epidural steroid injections (aka ESIs) are extremely common in the U.S. They are indicated predominantly for *radiculopathy*, or on rare occasion for postherpetic neuralgia (related to *shingles*). *Radiculopathy* is a disorder that affects the function of a nerve root. The effects of radiculopathy can include any of the following:

- Numbness
- Weakness
- Loss of reflexes
- Paresthesias (tingling, pricking, and burning)
- Leg or arm pain (aka *radicular* pain)

A patient feels or notices a *predictable and defined* pattern with radiculopathy; the patterns are referred to as *dermatomes*. (see Figure 5) A physical examination can indicate this disorder, but an MRI (magnetic resonance imaging) may allow the physician to correlate the symptoms with the anatomy to enable a more definitive diagnosis.

When a physician evaluates a suspected radiculopathy, it is common also to order an *electromyogram (*EMG*) and nerve conduction studies (*NCS*)*. These studies further clarify nerve irritation, but can be quite uncomfortable for most patients. The EMG measures the electrical activity of muscles at rest and during contraction. The NCS measures how well and how fast the nerves can send electrical signals. These studies give some additional information to the physician in conjunction with the patient history, physical exam and *appropriate* imaging. These can be uncomfortable procedures and may or may not be helpful in determining an accurate diagnosis.

One must remember that **not all "shooting" pain is radiculopathy**. Unfortunately, there are many cursory examinations done in the medical field when there is limited time with the patient. A tight hamstring may be misconstrued as *radicular pain* especially if a thorough exam is not done. *Pain radiating or referring to other areas* may not be related to *true* radicular pain, but an epidural steroid injection may be prescribed anyway. Unfortunately, ESIs seem to be done on patients more empirically than most physicians are willing to admit. In other words, many patients with a *suggested yet unconfirmed* radiculopathy are frequently scheduled for ESIs. With poor selection of appropriate patients, it is no surprise that a significant percentage of those injections do not improve the patient's pain especially when it is not addressing the actual *cause* of the pain. Hence, **more epidural steroid injections are done than necessary**.

If a patient is experiencing *true* radiculopathy, then it is usually related to a herniated disc or a narrowing of the bony opening (foramen) through which the nerve root exits the spinal column. On occasion, pain can be attributed to non-mechanical reasons such as inflammatory chemicals released from a disc into the area of the spinal nerve. Rarely, the cage or column where the spinal cord lives

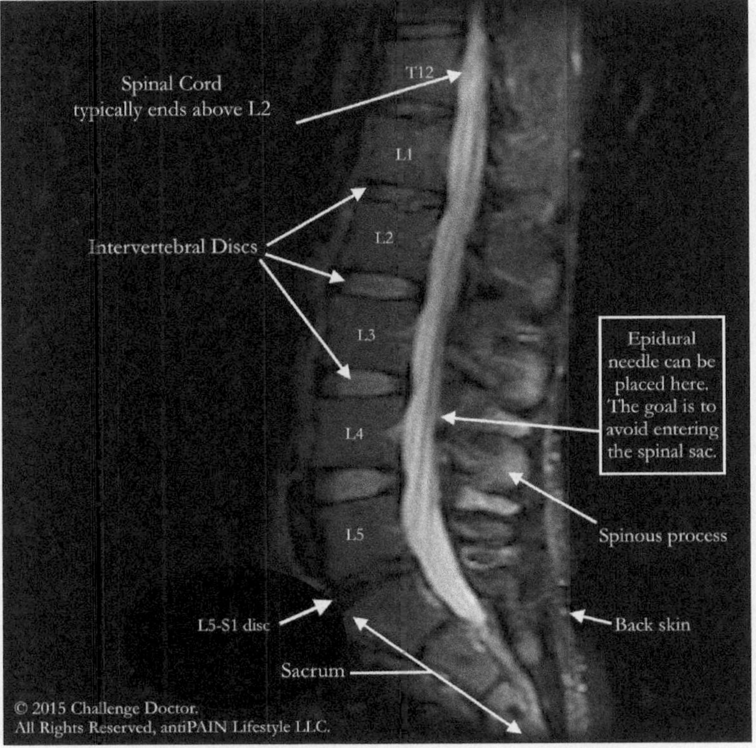

Figure 6: A standard epidural steroid injection places the numbing medicine and/or steroid near the area or nerve in question, but *outside of the spinal sac*. This illustration shows an injection into the lumbar spine, which is the typical location used for epidurals during childbirth and for low back pain with *radiculopathy*. However, epidural needles can be placed anywhere along the spine up to the low neck depending on the location of perceived pain. The higher up the spine, the higher the risk for *entering the spinal sac (severe headache possible) or injuring the spinal cord (numbness, weakness, paralysis)*.

can become so narrow due to bony or soft tissue growth that it can squeeze the spinal cord causing changes to the nerves supplying the arms or more commonly, the legs—this is called *spinal stenosis*.

Epidural steroid injections must be carefully monitored when a patient uses blood thinners or is a poorly controlled diabetic. Bleeding and possible paralysis can occur with too much bleeding against the spinal cord. This is why **blood thinners must be discussed** in order to evaluate if and how long the blood thinner should be discontinued around the time of the planned epidural injection. **Diabetics must be watched closely**, as life-threatening elevated glucose levels can result from an injected steroid. Careful consideration of the steroid dose and close management of a diabetic patient's glucose must take place.

An epidural needle is typically slightly bigger than a needle used for a spinal, but the needle is targeted to an area *just outside the spinal sac* to place the medications. (see Figure 6) The space targeted by the epidural needle can have many epidural veins, which can lead to excessive bleeding if blood thinners are used or if a bleeding disorder exists.

Spinal Cord Stimulators

Spinal cord stimulators can be used for a variety of pains, including CRPS-related arm pain or low back pain with associated leg pain. These devices are usually placed on a trial basis before a permanent placement is done. In essence, with mild or no sedation, an epidural-like procedure is done by advancing one or more leads via a needle *into the space just outside the spinal sac*. The leads are skinny, specialized cords that have multiple internalized metallic contacts to allow various programming configurations to **mask the pain with a tingling sensation** (aka *paresthesia*); however, there are newly developed spinal cord stimulators approved by the Food and Drug Administration that function *without* tingling sensations.[75] The trial procedure includes a representative from one of the few spinal cord stimulator companies in the United States who will assist the physician and the patient with localizing and programming the stimulation. Use of more than one lead depends on several factors and increases the cost of the overall procedure.

Although patients are typically given a medication that makes it difficult to recall interactions during the procedure, **patient cooperation and feedback are essential to determine the best location of the lead or leads**. After the leads are positioned in the ideal location to obtain tingling sensations in the area of prior pain complaints, they are temporarily secured with tape to the skin and connected to an external battery. The spinal cord stimulator representative then helps the patient with programming the device and how to use any available remote controls. Afterward, the patient's objective is *typically* to assess the amount of function gained and to determine if roughly 50 percent or more pain relief has occurred over the following three to five days. The length of time can vary but infection from a temporary lead is a valid concern over time.

The temporary spinal cord stimulator lead is usually removed in the doctor's office. If permanent placement is warranted and desired by the patient, then it is done under some level of sedation and sometimes under general anesthesia. Patient cooperation is ideal for permanent placement but if the physician is comfortable with the desired lead location, then patient interaction may not be necessary. In a permanent placement, the leads are placed the same way but with a larger incision to allow the leads to be anchored to deeper tissues. This allows the entire system to be contained within the body to avoid infection and for long-term stability. The battery is typically placed in the back or buttocks via a deep skin pocket made with an incision. In order to connect the battery to the secured leads, a tunnel is created deep in the skin to allow the leads from the epidural space to travel to the battery location.

Some newer versions of the spinal cord stimulators are MRI-friendly, but the others are contraindicated for MRI machines, which is a downside for future imaging of other medical issues. Aside from the anesthesia and surgical risks of this minor surgery, spinal cord stimulator leads can sometimes move from their original position requiring additional re-programming or surgery. Or perhaps, the pain relief may decrease over time, which may be due to the *neuroplasticity* or changeability of the nervous system.

Implantable Pain Pumps

An implantable pain pump is another minor surgery option to address a variety of pains. These can be permanently placed within a patient especially if the pain has been managed by high doses of opioids that created undesirable side effects, such as severe constipation or mental impairment. By the time a patient receives a pain pump, many other invasive procedures *may* have been tried without acceptable improvement—but not all patients are given extensive conservative options. The patient receiving a pump is *usually* under general anesthesia in a face down or side down position. This position allows the pain physician to *access the spinal cord sac* with an *epidural-like* needle inserted in the middle of the spinal column with an approach similar to the *spinal* procedure described earlier. Once a small amount of spinal fluid is recognized, a catheter is advanced *through* the needle and *into the spinal sac*. The needle is removed, and a deep skin pocket for the pain pump or medication reservoir is fashioned via an incision in the back or abdomen. A tunnel is made beneath the skin connecting the catheter in the middle of the back to the pain pump to keep the system contained within the body. Careful management of the local anesthetic, opioids, or other medications within the pump is necessary, and refills are typically done every one to three months. Because it is a piece of equipment, there is always a chance of malfunction.

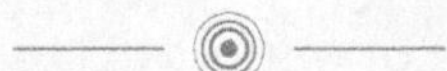

It is helpful to have an idea what it costs for these more invasive procedures. In a current surgery center that offers unusually *transparent* pricing for patients paying cash for pain procedures, here are the total costs for the facility *and* the physician fee[76]:

- Cervical epidural steroid injection: $1,100
- Lumbar epidural steroid injection: $700
- Lumbar sympathetic nerve block: $1,580
- Stellate ganglion block: $1,100

The fees charged by most hospitals, surgery centers, and physicians vary widely and can be derived from the "game" of guessing what the insurance company will pay, which varies as well. It is not easy even for a physician to get a transparent assessment of reimbursement prior to billing for the procedure. For example, the cost for a *spinal cord stimulator* could be about $30,000 for Medicare patients. This includes the cost of the medical device, the physician who implants it, and the surgery center fee. For private insurance patients, the cost could be closer to $57,000. These costs do not include the maintenance visits, which could be $5,000 to $20,000 per year—assuming that there are:

- *No* migration or movement of the leads to an ineffective location
- *No* infections
- *No* bleeding
- Consistent pain relief

This is also assuming that all opioid use was weaned off around the time that the spinal cord stimulator was implanted, which does not happen for all patients. Often, pain patients with spinal cord stimulators remain on their oral pain medications indefinitely, which increases costs and associated risks. Occasionally patients can rely strictly on the spinal cord stimulator for pain relief. If a patient is unsatisfied with the stimulator over time, then there is the option of paying even more money to remove and throw away the $13,000 to $19,000 piece of equipment![77]

The bottom line is that there are some high costs associated with dampening the pain signals using the above procedures, which may not be addressing the definitive *cause* of pain. Can they help bridge someone out of pain to increase function? Yes, I have personally performed these procedures during my medical training and some people improved, but many patients kept returning with pain. Some would argue that physicians with a special interest in pain might have incomplete knowledge of how to treat pain, especially back pain.[78] In many cases, I must agree with that. Unfortunately, as Dr. Karel Lewit, a Czech Republic Manual Therapist (1916-2014) quoted, "He who treats the *site* of pain is lost!"

Indeed, pain physicians are targeting the *perceived site* of pain with injections—yet, they are not the sole answer to helping pain patients.

CHAPTER 10

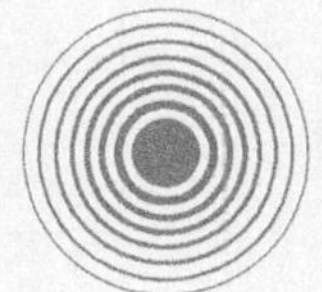

The Good, The Bad, and The Ugly of Major Surgery

Numerous pain sufferers describe being driven to have surgeries that only ended up exacerbating their pain and causing greater disability.
—**Institute of Medicine**, *Relieving Pain in America*

Major surgery, such as spine surgery, is one of the riskiest approaches for non-emergent, chronic, non-cancer pain. It violates the intrinsically amazing aspects of the body.

There are times when surgery can be helpful, as when treating:

- a growing mass creating radiculopathy
- a large primary cancerous mass—especially if obstructing vital organs
- a growing or large blood clot compressing the spinal cord
- true radiculopathy from a herniated disc that is causing neurologic changes such as *foot drop* (i.e., cannot move ankle to lift toes off the ground)

Incredibly skilled and brilliant surgeons *can save lives and help patients* with serious issues. This is the **good** side of surgery.

The **bad** side of surgery is that sometimes it *does not help with pain*, but it is still touted as the best hope for so many patients *before* putting them through conservative measures such as intensive physical and cognitive therapy.[79,*] Ironically, I have met many patients who have had lumbar fusions but still had pain after the fusion. Then they return to the operating room to have the hardware removed. The question is whether the patient required that hardware in the first place. Moreover, once the hardware is gone, there is little offered to the patient beyond more surgery, medications, and injections.[80,81,82,83]

Patients' bodies are forever changed by surgery, whether inconsequential or profound. In most cases, the body will respond to the trauma of surgery and heal. However, when pain, as cryptic as it can be sometimes, is the primary reason to pursue surgery, there better be a darn good reason for the patient to undergo those risks! (see Figure 7) I know plenty of pain medicine physicians and surgeons who would avoid back surgery like the plague if they were the patients. *That should make you hesitate at least for a moment.* I am *not* convinced by the literature or from patients I have seen that spinal fusion is the most appropriate or most functional approach to *nonspecific* low back pain (*back pain with no neurologic concerns and/or no obvious cause*). Besides, a patient will likely be a repeat customer to a surgeon once the segment above or below a fusion surgery starts changing its appearance. The mechanics of the spine is altered above and below the fusion, which minimizes *normal* motion and is likely to cause future problems.[84,85]

Down the road after fusion surgery, it is quite easy for the physician and the patient to believe that radiographic changes combined with *worsening* pain are proof that those changes are responsible for the unresolved or increasing pain. However, there are real surgery and anesthesia risks when assuming that

---

* *Cognitive (behavioral) therapy*—treatment that incorporates multiple methods such as enhancing one's awareness of thoughts, instilling motivational self-talk, minimizing self-defeating thought, or changing maladaptive beliefs about pain in order to help minimize the intensity of pain. Addressing fear-avoidance behaviors is part of this therapy.

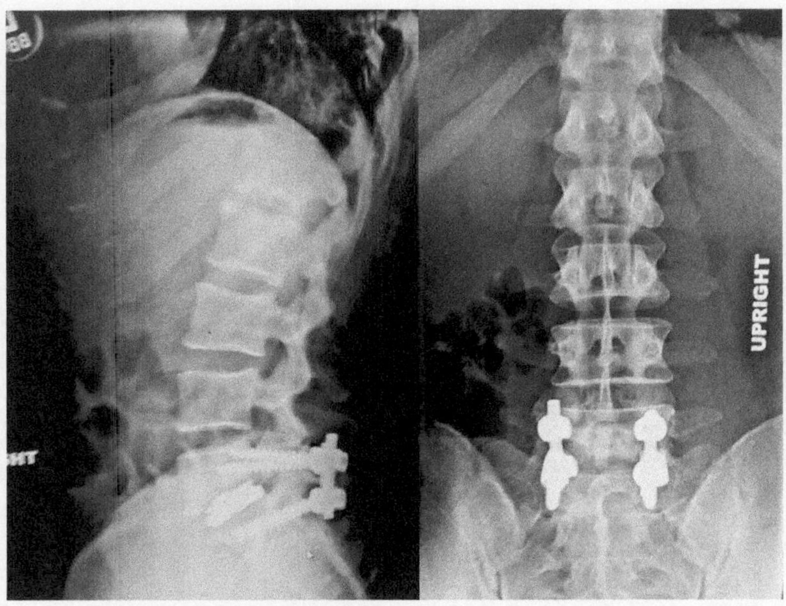

Figure 7: This highly functional patient had back pain with no neurologic deficits and capable of working out at a gym squatting hundreds of pounds not long before surgery. With chronic low back pain complaints, the patient chose to undergo fusion between the 5th lumbar vertebra (L5) and the sacrum (S1), per the surgeon's recommendations. The pictures here were taken not long after surgery. A disc spacer was also placed and appears white in this image between the bones containing hardware. The patient admitted that the pain experienced *after* surgery was more than anticipated and the surgery may have been a mistake; time will tell. *Permission for photos obtained from patient.*

radiographic changes correlate with pain necessitating surgery. The surgical risks include failure to fix or address the problem, new or worsening pain, bleeding with a possible transfusion, allergic reactions, infection, airway complications, nerve injuries, cardiac events, lung complications, and even death. **Even under the best circumstances, bad things can happen during surgery.** To top it off, if the patient is not practicing healthy habits or is unhealthy, then chances are increased, as small as they may be, for adverse outcomes during or after any surgery.

There are many surgeries being performed for pain, especially on the spine. However, even orthopedic surgeons and neurosurgeons are admitting that comprehensive and intensive rehabilitation with cognitive behavioral therapy (CBT) has similar outcomes as lumbar fusion surgery. Cognitive behavioral therapy is a form of psychotherapy, which addresses thoughts and feelings that may be counterproductive to dealing with issues in life, including pain. Orthopedic surgeons and neurosurgeons had this to say recently regarding the lumbar fusions they perform:[86,87]

> *There is Level II evidence to support lumbar fusion over traditional physical therapy alone, but that benefit is not present when fusion is compared with a more intensive physical therapy program with cognitive therapy.*

They admit that patients with intractable low-back pain *without stenosis or spondylolisthesis* "remain a difficult problem with many unanswered questions." In their words…

> *…further investigation will be necessary to improve the diagnostic capabilities of identifying the origin of pain in this patient population. With improved diagnostic capabilities, intervention can be directed at the primary pathological process.*

Apparently, there are back surgeries being performed that are neither relieving pain or shown to be superior to aggressive, noninvasive approaches. **Ultimately, the diagnostic accuracy of determining "why" someone has back pain is woefully lower than desired—leading to many unnecessary risks. "Diagnosing" back pain is truly a medical challenge.**

The challenge has been there for years, even before MRIs were available. In a landmark article on correlating herniated discs with *sciatica* by the surgeons Mixter and Barr in 1934, one of the authors replied to comments in a discussion with the New England Surgical Society:[88]

There have been two or three cases, which I have operated on expecting to find the lesion and in which I have had a negative exploration, and those we have not included in this presentation today because it seemed to us to confuse the picture. It is a difficult diagnosis to make and we have been wrong several times.

The author recognized the difficulty and uncertainty involved in understanding the cause of the sciatica *without* serious red flags. He noted that patients could get better with conservative treatment without surgery. Yet, one of the several conclusions of the study was that a herniated disc "…should be borne in mind in the study of certain orthopedic conditions, particularly in those cases which do not respond to appropriate treatment." He then elaborated on patients receiving surgical fusion:

I may be wrong, but it seems to me if you have given such cases fixation and they still have pain, then you have a right to go ahead and do a laminectomy. I think fusion should be combined with operation where there is any question of the unstable spine, and I believe that a ruptured disc may be unstable.

It is clear in 2015 that NOT *all* ruptured discs are "unstable." Drs. Mixter and Barr may have helped numbers of *symptomatic* patients with significant *red flags*, but the 1934 study led to more *surgical fixation* of spines and more *mental fixation* on discs as the problem. It is no surprise that *over 80 years later* patients can be concerned or easily swayed to surgery merely by pain and MRI findings, with which they are not familiar.

There is enormous impatience and underutilization of conservative approaches early on with pain, even though the cost of comprehensive pain programs is undeniably less expensive than traditional medical treatment, which includes surgery. The reality is there is little financial incentive for surgeons, surgery centers, or hospitals to promote conservative approaches. The irony is that third party payers more easily reimburse for numerous invasive approaches and less for comprehensive pain programs. This creates a frustration and a challenge for patients and physicians to find the most appropriate, conservative, and integrated care.[89]

Some of the largest financial costs for back pain can come from surgery. Here are the costs for the facility and the physician fee from a current surgery center that offers transparent pricing for patients *paying cash*:[90]

- One-level neck fusion surgery with hardware: $18,960
- Lumbar laminectomy: $9,900
- Lumbar microdiscectomy: $8,855

If *insurance* is involved, then here are possible costs *at a hospital*:

- Lumbar microdiscectomy: $20,000-$50,000
- Lumbar discectomy: $15,000-$75,000
- Lumbar fusion: $75,000-$100,000+

Although the insurance company is billed a certain amount, they tend to pay less than the billed amount. Based on a 2009 insured patient's lumbar fusion surgery, which required a three-day hospital stay:[91]

- Hospital billed insurance $93,000, but received $61,000
- Surgeon billed for $19,400, but received $6,000
- Anesthesiologist billed for $5,000, but received $2,000
- Although $117,400 was billed, only $69,000 was received in payment

Fifty-eight percent of the amount billed toward the insurance company still cost the patient and society $69,000—big moneymaker, but only $8,000 went to the two physicians from that $69,000. The hospital and medical device companies received the larger payout.

Unfortunately, the cost did not guarantee pain relief, and many times surgery does not change a patient's pain or quality of life. Sometimes the pain goes away, because the surgery addressed the real problem. Sometimes psychologically, it was aggressive enough to make the patient *believe* it would help—also known as *placebo*. Perhaps the pain was going to resolve on its own. Maybe the manipulation or stretching of the connective tissue during the surgery helped. (see Figure 8) Maybe the surgery gave the patient more support, expectation, and motivation to do the physical therapy more intensely and consistently than before the surgery. It is difficult to prove the "why."

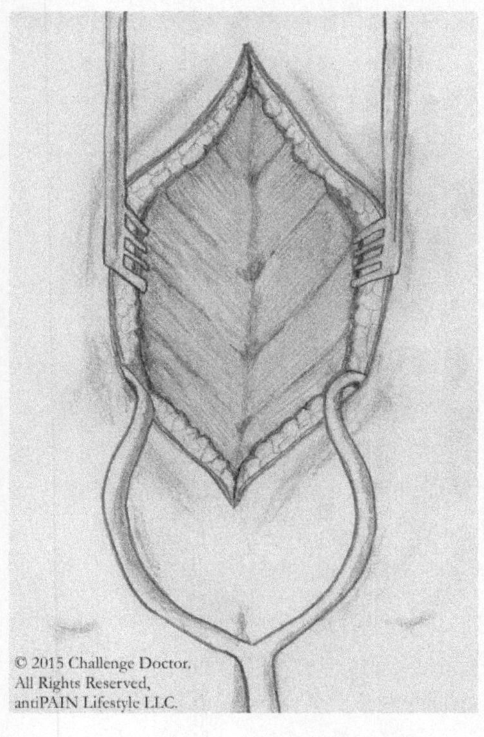

Figure 8: This is a depiction of instruments retracting skin/ connective tissue/fat during an approach for lumbar (low back) spine surgery. What is exposed underneath in this image are the muscles/ connective tissue. At the midline are the "bumps" or impressions made by the underlying tips of the spinous processes, which are the most superficial aspects of the bony spine. Retraction of the tissues allows for further dissection and exposure of the spine throughout the surgery, such as during a lumbar fusion.

The power of *placebo* can apply to any pain, including knee pain. As early as 2002, there was a controlled trial performed on 180 elderly men diagnosed with osteoarthritis knee pain. They were divided almost equally into three groups. The first group received three incisions around the knee, but no surgery was done inside the knee. The second group had fluid flushed within the knee, but minimal to no cleanup or debridement of tissues was done. The third group had extensive debridement of the meniscus and smoothing out of internal knee surfaces. After one year, there was *no* difference in knee pain or self-reported function among all groups. In fact, at various points within that year, the *observed function* of the men who received *extensive debridement* was *significantly worse* than those in the placebo group.[92] Results such as these certainly make surgery a more questionable option. Thus, consideration of surgery not related to a limb- or life-threatening situation is worth some patience, research, and multiple opinions.

The **ugly** side of surgery is that some serious consequences can occur. Infection, bleeding, and nerve injury are just a few surgical risks. Of course, anesthesia risks are implied including heart risks, airway risks, and allergic reactions, etc. Infection is a concern, especially in diabetics, alcoholics, or anyone with a compromised immune system, but it can happen to anyone. When a foreign body is involved with the infection, such as plates, screws, or cages inserted into or onto the spine, then that hardware is usually pulled out of the body when the infection is cleared out. This could create an extremely long recovery process with repeat procedures. As for bleeding, there are large vessels (e.g., aorta, inferior vena cava) that sit in front and to the side of the spine that must be avoided. With the various approaches and instrumentation used for spine surgery, there can sometimes be additional nerve injury to the nerve of concern or nearby nerves. On rare occasion, this can lead to numbness, pain, or inability to move certain parts of an extremity.

Through multiple studies and reviews, it is quite clear that surgery has a higher cost and a higher risk of complications versus comprehensive and intensive rehabilitation.[93] There are many surgeons who staunchly defend back surgery for the pain patients they do help; yet, general surgeons may be equally offended by the assertion that some of their patients could lose weight conservatively without their gastric surgery. By cutting on or altering the body, there is a chance of causing other problems. **Given the complexity of the body's integrated system, surgery is not the panacea for every pain, especially back pain. If there are no red flags, then surgery as a first option makes very little sense.**

I am always alarmed by how many patients, upon my nonchalant questioning, reveal NO conservative attempts at improving their condition prior to heading back to the operating room. As an example, patients who were mildly obese and with only borderline medical issues were undergoing body-altering gastric bypass surgery despite admitting that they did not do any guided exercise or dietary changes in their life prior to going "under the knife." The physician and the patient in those circumstances believe or convince themselves that surgery is the only way to accomplish the goal. As for pain patients pursuing injections or non-emergent back surgery, many interviewed patients also had minimal to no conservative approaches, such as manual, movement, or behavioral therapy. Yet, surgery was pursued *initially*? According to a surgeon, Dr. Wilco Peul, "Preventing surgery is a goal we should all chase."[94]

Don't confuse surgery as good for all, bad for all, or ugly for all. There is a time and a place for surgery. The risks and benefits should be clearly understood, but they are not always explained thoroughly. The explanation is dependent on the surgeon's thoroughness, integrity, and time—and, of course, *patient questions*. The medical system may balk at slowing down the day for a busy physician, but questions should be answered. Just like asking for a translation from someone speaking another language, patients should ask for a simpler explanation of the surgical plan if not understood. Patients should feel as comfortable as possible with a surgery decision. Many patients *can* benefit from *some* types of surgery. **Yet, if there is no emergent reason for surgery, then pursuing conservative approaches for pain with the mind and body should be discussed initially.** It breaks my heart to hear patients tell me, *"If I knew then, what I know now, then I would not have had surgery."* Sadly, I have had *many* patients admit this to me… and I believe them.

CHAPTER 11

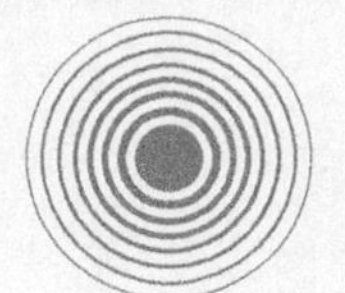

Limitations of Evidence-Based Medicine

Medicine is a science of uncertainty and an art of probability.
—William Osler

Sometimes the media, attorneys, or medical professionals will speak of evidence-based medicine, but this is a new term. *Evidence-based medicine* (EBM) within the medical field was formally introduced in the late 1900s[95] and is defined as "the conscientious, explicit and judicious use of current best evidence in making decisions about the care of individual patients."[96] Yet, the formal scientific method began several centuries prior. Per the Oxford English Dictionary:

> *The scientific method is a method or procedure that has characterized natural science since the 17th century, consisting in systematic observation,*

measurement, and experiment, and the formulation, testing, and modification hypotheses.

That is quite a mouthful, but it is not always easy to measure or test certain hypotheses with experiments or research. For example, running a controlled trial on the effectiveness of wearing *or not wearing* a parachute during free fall from hundreds of feet in the sky would not be approved.[97]

However, research that *is* approved can still be fabricated, contradictory, conflicted, or poorly done.[98] The human body is complex; therefore, it is somewhat foolish of us to think we can reduce our complicated bodies into simplistic processes. There is nothing about us that is simple. We have a long way to go despite the advances that continue in medicine. While great medical research is available, physicians do not always have the time nor do they always know about new research, especially when a barrage of studies is released on a daily basis.

Research is usually designed to compare an intervention or surgery to an *appropriate conservative treatment*. What does *appropriate conservative treatment* really mean? If physical therapy was used, then there may be multiple techniques and approaches with which to treat the patient. Thus, *appropriate conservative treatment* is somewhat vague and does not guarantee the same quality of treatment across all patients. As a result, the numbers calculated from that study may not be accurate as to the effectiveness of a particular intervention.

Nowadays, physicians are expected to guide their practice by evidence-based medicine, which is based upon a select *population* of patients, not the *individual* patient. There are plenty of things that physicians learn during training that are evidence-based, but they can be discarded or rarely used in clinical practice if deemed unhelpful or not applicable to a particular patient. On the contrary, it is insensible to discard or to minimize the lower risk yet potentially helpful options for a patient's problem merely because of a lack of EBM or based solely on low insurance reimbursement. It remains challenging to convince my medical colleagues who are living with pain that there are other ways of assessing or treating it beyond what is offered or proven by EBM. It is easy for physicians to justify what should be done for a patient simply because it has always been done that way or it is what they have learned. Because each person is unique and EBM does not always fit the *individual*, physicians must keep their focus on the *patient*. Clinical experience helps the physician decide what is in the best interest of the patient and whether evidence-based medicine applies to that individual.

Taking EBM a step further and creating treatment *algorithms* or "cookbook" approaches may seem to be efficient and safe in some settings, but not necessarily for the chronic pain patient. However, pain *business* models with a high volume of patients would likely prefer otherwise.[99]

If there was solid evidence that the way physicians are doing things in a traditional pain practice was very effective for the patient, then algorithms would be more acceptable. However, running patients through a clinic as if they are on a conveyer belt is ignoring some of the most important aspects of each patient's needs, which are to be heard and fully evaluated. A holistic approach by the physician to evaluate the multiple facets of each patient's life is not possible solely with de-personalized algorithms and brief office visits. Thus, **evidence-based practices and algorithms should merely be a guide for the patient's unique situation but never the prevailing drivers to do a procedure in chronic pain medicine**. There is just too much to be learned about pain for us to make concrete and unyielding statements. For now, the patient and the physician must be accepting of some uncertainty during the individualized pursuit of pain resolution or improvement.

Evidence-based medicine has its place but some conservative methods with weaker evidence may be just what a patient needs. Similar to how physicians can minimize or dismiss pain complaints because they cannot see it, it is common for physicians to dismiss therapies that are not strongly supported by EBM. If a physician does not appreciate other options as real possibilities to help with pain, then those avenues do not exist as alternatives—especially if the benefits are difficult to explain. However, if it is low-risk and low-cost, then it may be reasonable to review the possibilities of a trial with that patient. Trial and error with risky and expensive surgery that has a 50-50 chance of helping is not wise in my opinion. I am not supporting quackery. If a health professional has wisdom gained from personal experience or the experience of others about *low*-risk options, then it may be a reasonable place to start if it is in the best interest of a willing patient.

Throughout history, there have been instances of ideas running counter to the conventional wisdom of the day but later proven true by one or more brave souls willing to challenge the system. We all remember how everyone used to think the world was flat! It would be ludicrous for an adult today to think otherwise. In medicine, there used to be a lack of appreciation for gluten sensitivity in many women, which led to their psychiatric evaluation; now there is some science to support that patients can have abdominal pain secondary to sensitivity to gluten. Weight gain was once thought to be controlled exclusively by diet and exercise; now researchers have discovered the importance of sleep for weight control. Finally, migraines and multiple sclerosis used to be viewed as mental issues needing psychiatric evaluation until disproved through research discoveries. As further perspective is gained in the pain world, I surmise that later generations will likely scoff at the means by which we are currently addressing pain as well.

The evidence to support EBM protocols in pain can be elusive. Pain, by its very nature, can be frustrating for clinicians to explain because the cause can be difficult to uncover with the current state of medical training. The diagnoses in pain medicine are usually symptom-oriented, e.g., low back pain; thus, imprecise when used as the basis for research. Imagine doing a cataract surgery study where all of the research subjects were selected for *decreased vision*, but not *cataract development*. The symptom of decreased vision could apply to any number of eye problems, not just cataracts. **To ensure better study outcomes, researchers need appropriate subjects with similar *causes* of their problems**. Only then can a direct apples-to-apples comparison be done. In the cataract surgery study, if everyone was selected based on *decreased vision* without confirming all test subjects actually had cataracts, then the percentage of subjects who had improved vision after the cataract surgery would be lower than if they all truly had cataracts. Better results are obtained when the physician can pinpoint the reason for the symptom. Giving the same surgery to multiple people with similar symptoms but different causes does not make much sense. You can now "see" how accuracy of a diagnosis can make a difference in not only patient results, but in a research study's results. Similarly, lumping low back pain patients together in one study does not differentiate the various *causes* of low back pain. It is no surprise that *strong* evidence for low back pain treatments is lacking.

In the world of medicine or health, there are constant attempts to dissect and understand different elements of the body through research. There are expectations that evidence-based medicine is used for every decision. "Do no harm" is the motto, but not every decision or action faces grave risk. Evidence can be used to inform physicians and patients, but it cannot be a thoughtless endeavor. Common sense is required. There are lives at stake and many other aspects of the patient that must be considered before blindly accepting EBM.

Many surgeries are being done today that do not have a great deal of evidence as to their effectiveness, but they are still being performed. Conversely, many medical professionals want strong evidence for rational, noninvasive, and low-risk options where no or little evidence currently exists. I'm puzzled as to why the default or emphasis is *not placed* on those lower risk options to avoid harm until there is convincing data that a riskier procedure is worth it.

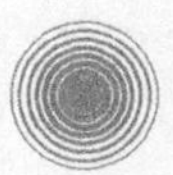

"Evidence can be used to inform physicians and patients, but it cannot be a thoughtless endeavor. Common sense is required."

Good sense, whether it is common or not, is not a bad thing to have in medicine. If something does not make sense, this should be discussed with the physician. **Reasonable options, even those with little direct evidence available currently, should be part of the discussion.** It is acceptable to question the reasoning for a physician's invasive options for pain, and at the same time push for treatment with the lowest risk. Patients benefit when they are active partners with their physicians. Self-advocating or collaborating with a patient advocate may be the best way to minimize the risk, assess the healing benefits available, and select the best course of treatment to reduce pain.

CHAPTER 12

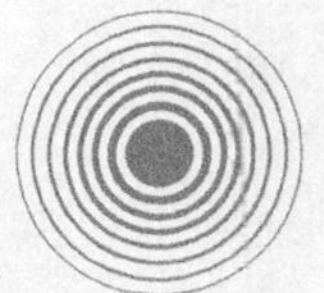

The Disk Risk: Understanding the Disc-onnect!

Sometimes people hold a core belief that is very strong. When they are presented with evidence that works against that belief, the new evidence cannot be accepted. It would create a feeling that is extremely uncomfortable, called cognitive dissonance. And because it is so important to protect the core belief, they will rationalize, ignore and even deny anything that doesn't fit in with the core belief.

—**Frantz Fanon**, *Black Skin, White Masks*

Herniated disc diagnoses are commonplace. So many friends, family members, colleagues, and patients talk about the "disc" in their back *giving them pain*. In most cases, a physician explained this likelihood based on a magnetic resonance image (MRI) interpretation.

Let's look at an example. (see Figure 9) How would you feel if this was your spine?

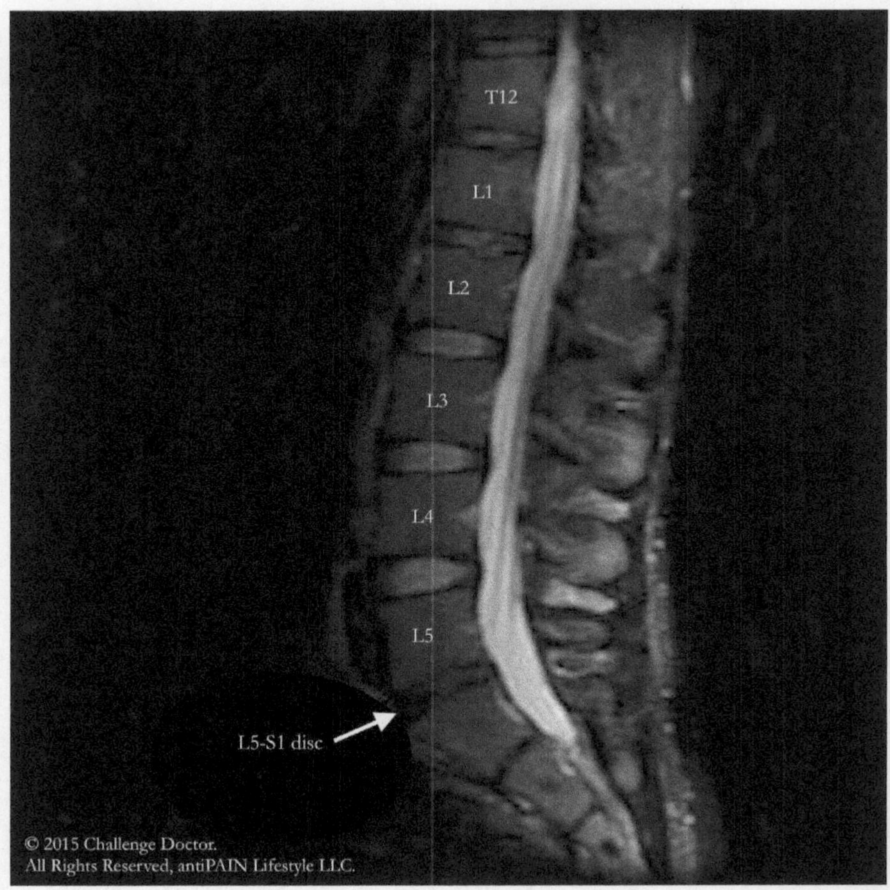

Figure 9: Adult lumbar spine MRI with no contrast used. This is a view from the side of the body.

It is a lumbar spine MRI of a typical adult patient and no contrast was injected into the patient's vein at the time of the study. Below is the assessment of the MRI. Please bear with the medical jargon.

The radiologist's findings were:

- The lumbar alignment is normal without fracture or subluxation. The vertebral body heights are maintained. Disc desiccation and mild loss of intervertebral disc height are noted at the L5-S1 level. The signal intensity of the bone marrow is normal.

- The conus medullaris terminates at L1 and is normal in caliber and signal intensity.
- L1-L2: Mild generalized disc bulge and mild bilateral facet hypertrophy with ligamentum flavum thickening result in no significant canal stenosis or neural foramina narrowing.
- L2-L3: Mild bilateral facet hypertrophy results in no significant canal stenosis or neural foraminal narrowing.
- L3-L4: A mild central disc bulge and moderate bilateral facet hypertrophy with ligamentum flavum thickening result in mild bilateral neural foraminal narrowing without canal stenosis. There is no definite exiting nerve root contact.
- L4-L5: A **moderate diffuse central disc bulge** and **moderate bilateral facet hypertrophy** with ligamentum flavum thickening result in mild bilateral neural foramina narrowing without canal stenosis. There is no definite exiting nerve root contact.
- L5-S1: **Mild circumferential disc bulge** and **moderate bilateral facet hypertrophy** with ligamentum flavum thickening result in no significant canal stenosis. **Mild to moderate bilateral neural foraminal narrowing** is noted with **near contact of the exiting L5 nerve roots.**
- The retroperitoneal soft tissues are unremarkable.

<u>**Overall Impression** *based on the findings above*</u>:

1. **Multilevel degenerative disc disease and facet hypertrophy of the lower lumbar spine** without evidence for lumbar spinal stenosis.
2. **Multilevel neural foramina narrowing, most notably at the L5-S1 level, mild to moderate bilaterally, with near contact of the exiting L5 nerve roots.**
3. *Correlation with the patient's symptomatology is suggested.*

The bolded areas are the suggested key findings of this MRI. Degenerative disc disease, bulging discs, and contact of nerve roots; it sounds pretty dire. Or is it?

A woman goes to her physician with some routine complaints. Her doctor examined her, and then gave her the bad news. "You appear to be suffering from degenerative hair and skin conditions. It must be painful." Shocked, the woman began to cry. Between sobs, she asked, "What can I do, doctor?" The doctor calmly replies, "Well, I would color my hair and get a good wrinkle cream if I were you."

In all seriousness, we all experience the aging process. We can see gray hair and wrinkles; they are visible and common. Yet, the *invisible aspects* of the human body are what can seem foreign, perplexing, and scary. When something sounds abnormal, like a herniated disc, patients often fear the worst. Here is the reality that most physicians know, but *most patients do not know*—**nearly everyone has a spinal "abnormality."**

If 100 patients with NO pain have an MRI done to evaluate the lumbar spine, anywhere from *29 to 76 of them would have disc herniations or other abnormalities*.[100] For patients presenting to a physician who actually have new back pain but no neurologic concerns, studies have shown pre-pain and post-pain MRI abnormalities reflect *age-related changes* and not the pain episode.[101] In other words, most patients who receive their first MRI assume that the radiology findings are directly related to their pain, but in actuality, there is no other MRI for comparison to prove whether that "abnormality" was there before or not. These simple yet profound studies started in the 1990s and continue today. These results are not surprising to most physicians, especially pain physicians. Despite this, patients are still being sent for MRIs and referred to surgeons when they do not have concerning neurologic signs or symptoms. When the answer to pain is not clear, the default is to offer referrals and studies, not reassurance.

The same logic applies to the neck. Another MRI study evaluated the cervical spines (necks) of 63 volunteers with NO pain.[102] Discs were degenerated or narrowed at one level or more in 25 percent of the subjects who were *less than* 40 years old. If older than that, almost 60 percent of the subjects had degenerative discs! **Just as skin and hair changes, so do the discs and bones of the spine. In other words, incremental changes due to aging or other stressors can alter the appearance of the body, but it does not always indicate pain or the "cause" of pain.**

Is it possible that patients and physicians are blaming the disc when it really is not the culprit? Absolutely. There is no doubt that simply prescribing surgery for a disc when there is NO nerve compromise (leading to leg pain, numbness, or weakness) does not make sense! There is limited value in the MRI for low back pain if there are no red flags.[103] In fact, MRI findings can encourage patients to worry about so-called "abnormalities" when they are not relevant to their pain.

Look at the following three charts to see how your age compares to the percentage of people **who have NO pain** but still have MRI spine abnormalities:[104]

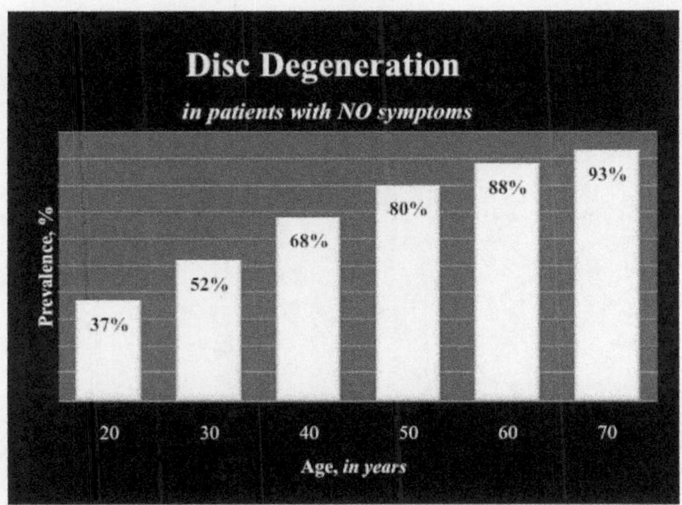

Modified from: W. Brinjikji et al, "Systematic Literature Review of Imaging Features of Spinal Degeneration in Asymptomatic Populations," Am J Neuroradiol 2014 Nov 27: 1-6. [Epub ahead of print] 2014© by American Society of Neuroradiology.

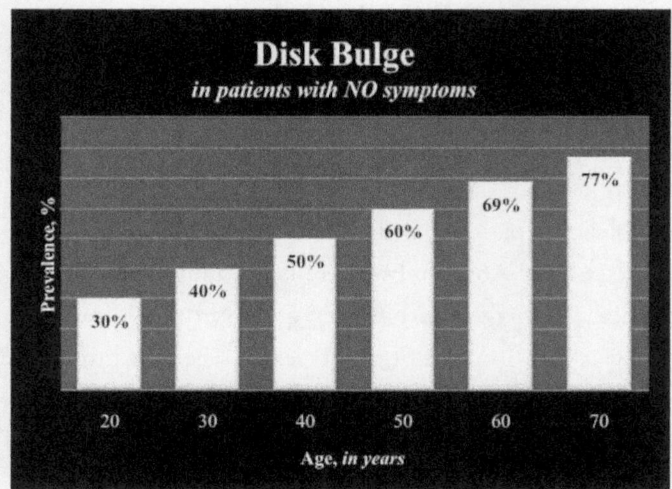

Modified from: W. Brinjikji et al, "Systematic Literature Review of Imaging Features of Spinal Degeneration in Asymptomatic Populations," Am J Neuroradiol 2014 Nov 27: 1-6. [Epub ahead of print] 2014© by American Society of Neuroradiology.

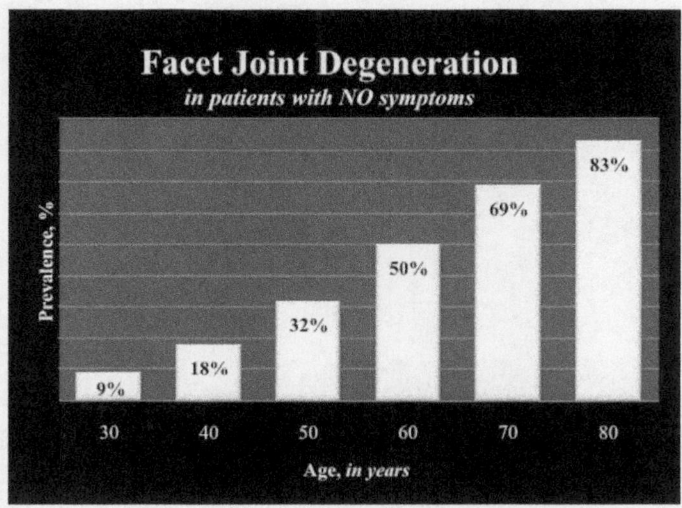

Modified from: W. Brinjikji et al, "Systematic Literature Review of Imaging Features of Spinal Degeneration in Asymptomatic Populations," Am J Neuroradiol 2014 Nov 27: 1-6. [Epub ahead of print] 2014© by American Society of Neuroradiology.

The "*disc*-onnect" comes from an assumption that disc abnormalities are the cause of someone's pain. As you can tell from the charts, there are high percentages of people who have abnormalities but no pain. Looking at the patient for red flags *first* versus looking at the disc or other common abnormality seems like a better approach. When the radiologist stated above, "*Correlation with the patient's symptomatology is suggested*," it is for a good reason.

Just as abnormalities in MRIs and X-rays do not guarantee they are correlated with pain, the opposite can be true. Normal MRIs can be found in patients with back pain. If the MRI is normal but the patient has pain, then the physician or patient can be confused and they may think that the pain is "all in their head." The physician may become frustrated at not having an answer. The patient is typically told it is not serious, but to the patient the pain is serious enough to bring them to the doctor's office. Not having answers can be very discouraging and depressing for the patient. The patient is the one experiencing the pain, whether the physician can see it or not.

However, if the MRI is abnormal, then a physician may assume that the cause of the pain is due to the "abnormality." In that case, the patient may be referred to a surgeon. For patients having associated pain, numbness, or weakness in the same nerve-related pathway as the nerve associated with the herniated disc indicated on the MRI, then surgery is likely to be a recommended course of treatment. If there is only back pain and no weakness, reflex changes, pain, or numbness, then the herniated disc or other abnormality is unlikely to be causing a serious problem. Whether surgery is offered will depend on the clinical presentation of the pain and the surgeon's level of conservatism. Unfortunately, there are more surgeries occurring than necessary. Why do I know this? Because I meet countless patients who still have the same or worse pain despite surgery.

There are limitations to what MRIs can show. For instance, MRIs are detailed structural snapshots while the patient is lying down and very still. If the patient's back pain occurs mostly while sitting or doing certain types of activities, the cause of the pain related to function or movement of the musculoskeletal or connective tissue is not perceived by a typical static MRI while lying down. There are some efforts to do more functional MRIs, but it is difficult to prove if the positioning or method of the MRI would make a difference.

As for the MRI shown earlier in this chapter, *it is mine*. I paid out-of-pocket (cash), and the radiologist only received information that I was a "39 year-old female with a history of low back pain." The irony is that I had NO pain at the time of the MRI. Remember, I had previous low back pain that prevented me from tying my own shoes, which was a similar complaint by the 35th president of the United States, John F. Kennedy.[105] However, unlike me, he was taken down an invasive treatment path without resolution. His journey with pain was an interesting one and if "not for a *back brace*, which held him erect, a third and fatal shot to the back of the head would not have found its mark."[106]

As for my MRI, it would have been so easy to blame any or all of the MRI findings as the cause of my low back pain; but there was no pain. Granted, if, in the future, the disc becomes more degenerated, then the vertebral bodies could compress, allowing the little *facet* joints behind them to cram together. This could lead to more squeezing on the nerve roots exiting the spinal column or pain at the facet joints. Yet, most of what I do to alleviate or prevent my pain has little to do with addressing the discs or joints directly.

Unfortunately, tests are often ordered out of concern for missing something or to appease a patient request because the patient knows someone who had that test done. In some respects, this mimics the overuse of antibiotics (which kill bacteria, not viruses) for viral infections because many patients expect medicine for every ailment. Physicians may comply even though they know better or as a "just in case" approach. Physicians understand that patients want solutions. Patients typically feel better when something is *done* versus only receiving reassurance that they will get better. Ironically, paying for that reassurance *versus unnecessary imaging and interventions* for low back pain could ultimately save a patient the cost of further pain, expenses, and suffering if an unwarranted and risky path is averted.

A pain patient without red flags, who has an MRI done anyway, may receive invasive procedures that give limited to no relief. Since most back pain resolves on its own within a couple of weeks, a wait-and-see approach is a better option;

otherwise, conservative options are a good start. Unnecessary MRIs can also cause patients to fixate on a so-called "abnormality," which may have no relevance to their pain. This leads to the next section emphasizing a unique situation that deserves a name unto itself.

CHAPTER 13

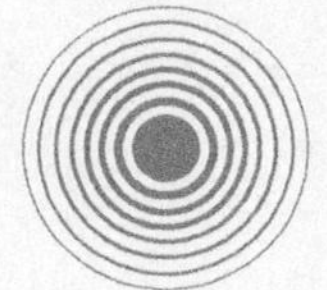

Are you Diagnocentric™?

People fall so in love with their pain, they can't leave it behind. The same as the stories they tell. We trap ourselves.

—**Chuck Palahniuk**, Novelist, *Haunted*

Anyone experiencing pain wants to know why the pain exists. At the very least, the person may just want help with making it go away. Either way, most patients are looking for a diagnosis and more importantly, a solution. Unfortunately, the business of medicine has arranged for those answers to be in the form of a diagnostic code, for insurance billing purposes. That diagnosis may be a description of your symptoms, like *lumbago*, or *low back pain*. The diagnosis just echoed your complaint; that's not very helpful.

What is the definition of *diagnosis*? It is the identification of the nature or *cause* of an illness or problem by *evaluating* the signs and symptoms—not *reiterating* the signs and symptoms. Yet, many "final" diagnoses are simply labeling the symptoms, not attempting to identify the causes.

The diagnosis of *complex regional pain syndrome* (CRPS) reflects a combination of *signs and symptoms*. As noted earlier in this book, CRPS usually involves one arm or leg or sometimes more than one extremity, but it can be anywhere and present with:

- Severe burning pain that is worse with a slight touch
- Skin changes of various colors
- Thin and shiny skin
- Arm or leg swelling
- Change in skin temperature to an arm or leg
- Nail and hair growth changes in that arm or leg

Other examples of syndromes that group a constellation of *symptoms* together are chronic fatigue syndrome or fibromyalgia.

Chronic fatigue syndrome is a debilitating and complex disorder characterized by intense fatigue for more than six months that does not improve with bed rest and may be worsened by physical activity or mental exertion. Fatigue typically interferes with daily activities or work. Other medical conditions are ruled out first prior to the diagnosis whereby at least four of the following symptoms are present:

- Post-exertion malaise (*lack of well-being*) lasting more than 24 hours
- Poor sleep
- Significant impairment of short-term memory or concentration
- *Muscle pain*
- *Pain in the joints* without swelling or redness
- *Headaches* of a new type, pattern, or severity
- *Tender* lymph nodes in the neck or armpit
- Frequent or recurring *sore* throat

Fibromyalgia is a disorder of unknown etiology characterized by *widespread pain* on both sides of the body, *abnormal pain processing*, sleep disturbance, fatigue, and often, psychological distress. There may be the following symptoms:

- Morning stiffness
- Tingling or numbness in hands and feet
- *Headaches*, including migraines
- Irritable bowel syndrome
- Sleep disturbances
- Problems with thinking and memory
- *Painful* menstrual periods and *other pain syndromes*

Although the diagnoses above are a description of symptoms, the actual diagnostic name may make some patients feel as if they can finally legitimize their pain or problems to themselves or others around them. Just because you are labeled with a diagnosis does not mean that the medical world understands *why* your symptoms exist or how to best deal with them. Ironically, most of the approaches to many of these poorly understood conditions involve optimizing one's lifestyle and/or pursuing alternative or complementary approaches with some traditional medications—in essence, harnessing the ingenuity of the human body by optimizing health.

Diagnoses are not always about the patient's symptoms. Sometimes the diagnosis is a reflection of a treatment that did NOT work, such as the important sounding: *failed back surgery syndrome* or *post-laminectomy syndrome*. Patients with either diagnosis received surgery in hopes of relief from a common and universal symptom, low back pain. However, the diagnosis does not explain anything except surgery was ineffective. Could it be the actual cause of the pain was misdiagnosed? For the patient, the diagnosis is meaningless. The pain is still present, and now the only relief offered may be injections, opioids, and further surgery…things the patient may have wanted to avoid. To add to the craziness, as you now know, neurosurgeons and orthopedic surgeons agree that intensive physical and cognitive therapy is just as effective as lumbar fusion.

A troubling aspect of insurance codes reflecting failed surgeries is they give the impression that everything was tried. This disempowering diagnosis can have patients believing they must accept and live with unresolved back pain and take medications for the rest of their lives. It is a disservice by physicians to limit options, to limit any hope, or to accept such descriptive diagnoses as appropriate or accurate. Granted, there are times when vague diagnoses such as "low back pain" are used during the course of "working up" or figuring out what is wrong or what helps the patient. If health care providers do not know why the patient has pain, then further assessment, research, or other resources should be pursued. Unfortunately, third-party payers such as insurance companies or worker's compensation systems hinder physicians by eventually restricting patient access to conservative or long-term treatments since there is limited money to go around. The reality is that it takes collaborative and consistent medical efforts or treatments to make headway for these challenging pain patients.

It is true that all health care professionals are capable of misdiagnosis or over-treatment with invasive or risky options. Each diagnosis, whether right or wrong, can lead down a long and windy road that may or may not help the patient.[107] Worst of all, if health professionals do not offer education or more conservative options to their patients, then they may be causing more harm. Physicians influence patients; thus, it is imperative that medical professionals give patients options that are more reasonable, regardless if they are not profitable. Most physicians will do this amid the stress of the current health care system situation, but physicians are a reflection of their education, training, experience, and personal development. Therefore, as always, there are different opinions. Those opinions may lead to different diagnoses or recommendations.

A diagnosis can have another chilling effect. It can lead the patient away from accepting personal responsibility for the problem. Since diagnoses are used to explain a situation, not always accurately, it gives patients something to latch on to as validation or as an excuse. Frequently, patients blindly accept a diagnosis without truly knowing the cause of their pain. This gives them little incentive to consider that *they* may be contributing to their own problem. Routine habits or behaviors may actually be contributing to or worsening their symptoms. A diagnosis makes it seem as if something happened *to* them, not because of something they did. Lifestyle *may not apply to all cases* but it should always be considered in the realm of possibilities. This is the situation I have termed **diagnocentricity**®:

> *The state of thinking of one's self as a diagnosis, without regard for the cause of the labeled medical condition and without effort to change the lifestyle that may lead to or worsen that condition. One could also describe a patient as being diagnocentric™.*

Most chronic ailments don't just show up overnight. A condition typically becomes chronic because of slow, subtle changes that occur over time. Because the body adapts over time, changes can be hard to see. This is not unlike a mother who sees her son every day, yet does *not* notice growth changes that are obvious to the child's aunt who only sees him twice a year. This is what can make a pain diagnosis so hard to believe, especially when no obvious recent trauma occurred. It could be due to concerning problems like cancer or less threatening issues like biomechanical or connective tissue changes that are too subtle to appreciate. Whatever the cause for the diagnosis, bodily changes can go unrecognized or barely perceived by human eyes until a problem arises or becomes chronic. Then, it can almost feel as if it's too late.

In some cases, it could be too late to bring the body back to its pre-chronic state but not always. Everyone has a genetic predisposition for various things. But it's how life is lived that will dictate which susceptibility genes turn on or turn off. Genes, just like the brain, are adaptable; that is, gene expression can change. The science behind this discovery is called *epigenetics*. A great example of altering gene expression is diabetes reversal. In the past, a diagnosis of Type 2 diabetes meant managing the disease with medications for the remainder of life. Today, we understand the causes behind diabetes more fully, and it is now possible to reverse this former life sentence in *most* cases, even if family genetics suggest otherwise. While this is exciting news, an even better way to manage diabetes is to keep from developing it in the first place. Just because diabetes may run throughout a family tree, understanding its causes, avoiding behaviors that fuel its development, and adopting positive eating and exercise behaviors may allow some family members to "dodge the diabetes bullet." How empowering! Optimizing and guiding genes in a positive and healthy direction, regardless of the diagnosis, can only help.

Of course, there are many people who will use a pain-related diagnosis, whether accurate or not, as a crutch, an excuse, or just a downright curse. Worst of all, **a "diagnosis" is a socially acceptable construct that can legitimize pursuing unnecessary and risky interventions.** Overutilization of health care comes at more than just a physical and psychological price, but a financial one as well. Just look at the United State's expenses on health care and the lousy payoff. Americans are not the healthiest. **By diagnosing and not educating or guiding patients down a path of rational and conservative care, those physicians are disempowering society and enabling a culture of passivity.** *Passivity does not lead to optimal health.* The immediate gratification of having something done by the health care system, like receiving opioids, injections, or surgery, can have consequences including allergic reactions, reversible or irreversible injury, further pain, despair, depression, distrust of health care providers, and the list goes on.

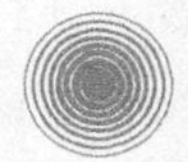

"Passivity does not lead to optimal health."

It is helpful to remember that a diagnosis is not a mathematical calculation as in Pain plus Diagnosis *X* always equals Treatment *Y*. The assumption that a diagnosis means a particular treatment should be pursued is not always accurate, but it depends on the diagnosis. That's where the physician comes in. Health care professionals may not know everything, but most of them will have enough knowledge, perspective, and skills to recognize issues that are concerning or guide pain patients down a better path for their health. The caveat is that the patient must be engaged in the conversation and not just be *obedient* to suggestions. There is always risk of being misguided down an unhelpful or risky path by caring providers. Reassessment of the situation and education are essential, and they cannot be accomplished without patient engagement.

The patient and physician must remember that some of the best health comes from *within*, not what is done *to* the patient. As much as I like making a difference in patients' lives, the variable response of patients and their behavior influences outcomes. The human body is truly amazing if given a chance and treated well. When it comes to lifestyle changes, sometimes patients need extra help to keep moving in the right direction consistently. Most health care providers *do* want to help, but the patient must be willing to put in real effort. For example, a patient suffering with weekly or monthly upper respiratory infections, but who continues to smoke a pack of cigarettes every day, stands little chance of truly getting better. Most of the time, humans can prevent bad health outcomes—or at least lessen the impact—by making smarter choices. Addictions like cigarettes can also stem from deeper reasons, such as anxiety and stress, which influence choices made.

Looking at the big picture of the patient's *biological, psychological, and social* situation is always better than isolating just the symptom. Called a *biopsychosocial* approach, it requires time, connection, communication, and an environment of collaboration. All of these factors are mostly sacrificed by the *business* of medicine, which leaves the patient disengaged and unlikely to make changes while the physician may be less fulfilled emotionally and intellectually. The patient and physician should *not just* focus on the so-called "diagnosis"—it's about the *whole* patient. Both will need to fight for doing the right thing to minimize the *diagnocentricity* associated with this country's *Paindemic*.

CHAPTER 14

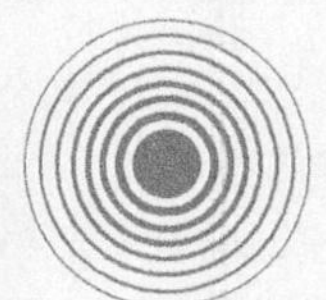

The Pain Patient Funnel

I think legislation needs to put an end to doctors profiting on businesses to which they can funnel patients – that is business, not medicine. If you try to call it medicine, then it is corruption. Without legislation, it will keep happening.

—Abraham Verghese, M.D.

In high volume pain practices, it is not uncommon for patients to go through an initial physical examination by a pain physician and then see a nurse practitioner or a physician assistant for the follow-up visits. If the pain practice follows *algorithms* or a predetermined set of steps for particular pain complaints, then the patient might only get to see the physician when interventions are scheduled. Yet, typically, there is little to no time for discussion with the pain physician on the day a procedure is performed, but this can vary by practice.

Patients in high volume practices have little interaction with their physicians, which is a detriment to the patients. Without consistent follow-up, including a reasonable exam by the physician, changes or subtleties may be easily missed. Too commonly, physician exams are brief and can merely consist of the physician lifting a leg off the table (see Figure 10) or straightening the leg while sitting (see Figure 11). Again, physical exams can vary greatly. These exams are testing for radiculopathy, which is usually followed by a suggestion for an epidural steroid injection but it may not be a *true* radiculopathy. Many times there are no further assessments to ensure that the patient's issue is not just tight hamstrings or other connective tissue issues.[108] I have witnessed quite a few patients, with tight hamstrings and no radiculopathy, who were told they have radiculopathy. Yet, these patients received one or more epidural steroid injections and do not understand why the steroids did not "work."

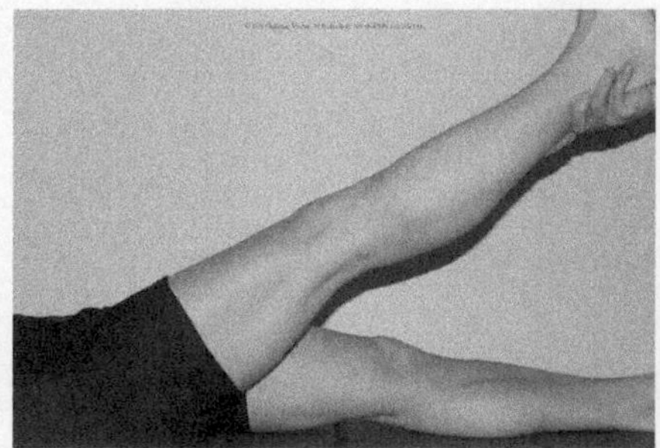

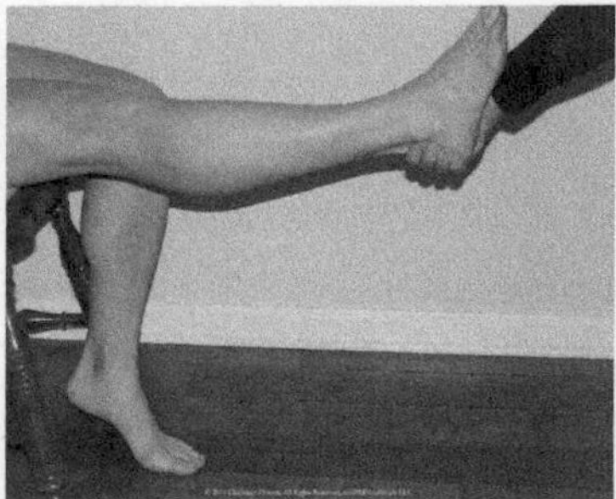

Figures 10 & 11: Leg tests to assess for radiculopathy. If this is the only thing that is done to assess low back pain and/or leg pain and there is no improvement, then have the physician explain or reassess. Otherwise, get a second opinion.

Regardless of the situation of health care, it is incredibly important to spend some time with patients with chronic pain. Inserting patients into an *algorithm* based on a few descriptions of pain during the history, one or two physical exam tests, and some imaging is not appropriate for all patients. It is important to have more extensive discussions of the patient's lifestyle, mechanism of injury, medical and surgical history, allergies, and social resources in addition to a thorough physical exam. *Some* patients have pain issues that are straightforward, but by the time most chronic pain patients see a pain medicine physician the problems are convoluted. In fact, they may already be on opioids adding another level of complexity to the situation. In addition, physicians relying on non-physician assistants *without* comprehensive pain training to do their follow-ups will likely perpetuate opioid refills and procedures.

Last time I checked, most patients do not want to be put on an *assembly line* without the physician re-examining or *connecting* with them. Pain is not just physical. Many psychological and emotional effects must be addressed while physical efforts are made to decrease or relieve the pain. It becomes increasingly important to look at the big picture to determine the real reason behind a patient's pain. This takes time and is why "pill mills" are notoriously poor at solving patient problems.

A pill mill is just like a "medical drive-through" with patients picking up prescriptions with little else offered. There is no real time to assess or help the patient with the *cause* of pain. Some patients swear by their medications and believe it may be the only way for them to function. Yet, many times there truly are better ways to deal with pain other than pills which carry addictive potential and a host of potentially serious side effects.

The pain patient funnel does not just refer to pills such as opioids, but procedures as well. There is a tendency to put many patients into a funnel with hopes that a particular procedure will help the patient's pain. It is a gamble. It is difficult to know who will feel better from certain injections, especially when the initial challenge of *diagnosing* pain correctly still has room for improvement. It is, therefore, no surprise that an enormous number of patients are receiving injections and medications with unremarkable outcomes. Only a small percentage will come out of the funnel pain-free. (see Figure 12)

There are physicians who spend time with their patients, perform thorough histories and physical examinations, and do not push interventions and pills first. I applaud them, for they are the exceptions. Pill mills or procedure farms, on the other hand, are volume-driven pain practices. They can be highly profitable to

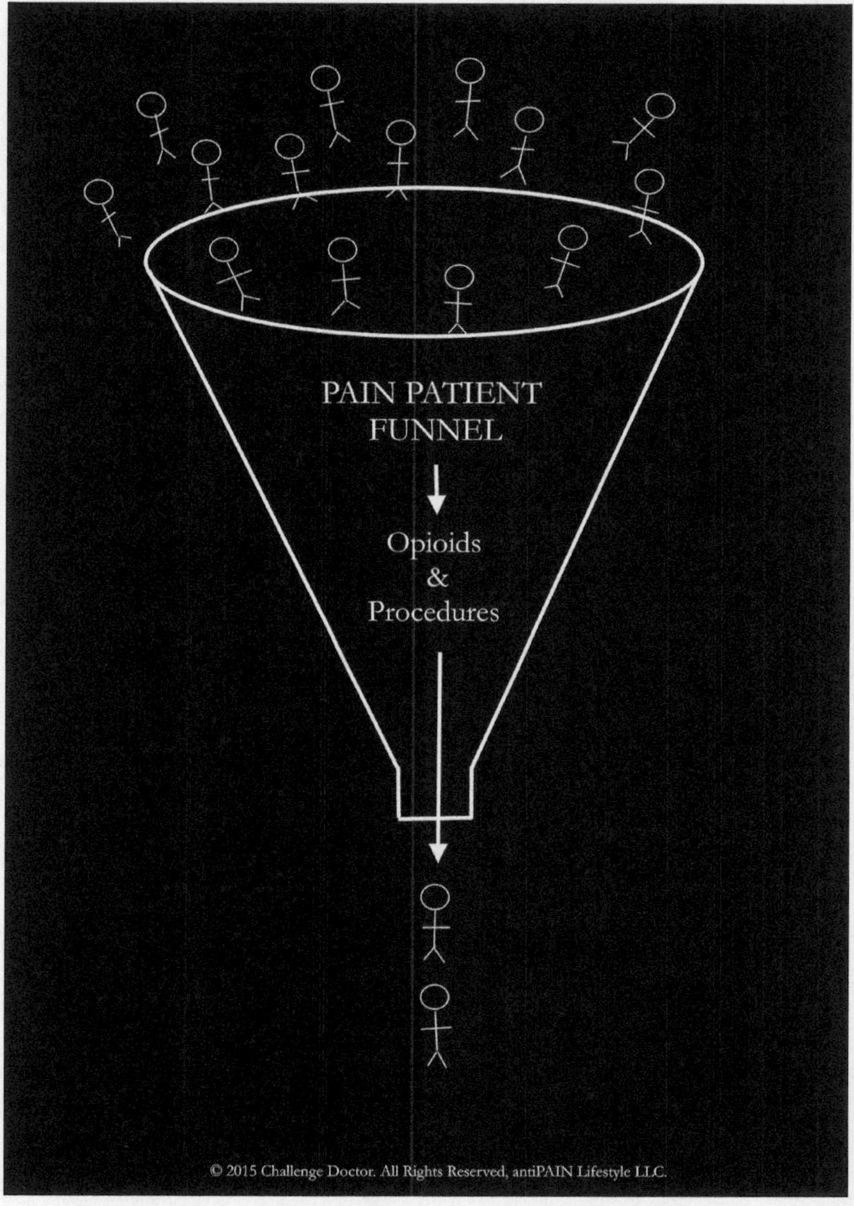

Figure 12: Many patients are offered opioids and invasive procedures with the "hopes" that their pain will get better. The reality is a small percentage of patients actually get rid of their pain by being passive in the pain patient funnel.

physicians and business executives in the world of health insurance, which has variable and fluctuating reimbursements. Due to limited time with the patient, the physicians in these practices take on an enormous risk, gather a lot of technical skill, but can be limited in their ability to be effective and helpful to the patients in the long run.[109] Patients may express brief gratification by getting what they *want or think they need* but patients are not educated and empowered to know how to do things for themselves. They are forever part of the pain patient funnel and are typically *frequent flyers* in many clinics or outpatient surgery centers. However, many patients do not want to be overly dependent on physicians to "fix" them through opioid use or increasingly risky procedures. At the same time, other patients are happy to assume passive roles regarding their health, which appears to be a reflection of the convenience-driven American society. Some patients may like the attention of the medical field, especially if "insurance covers it." However, physicians should always *try to educate and inform* patients as to the "what" and "why" of other approaches which may be more effective in treating pain in the end.

Ultimately, medical professionals should give patients the options or tools for helping themselves, whether patients choose to use them now or later. **Patients should have a choice to avoid the pain patient funnel and not be subjected to it unknowingly.** It is unbelievable how many patients do not realize there are other options out there beyond their own pain physician's treatments. Alternatives should be discussed or offered to patients whether it is financially beneficial to the health care professionals or not! This sounds idealistic, but deep down most physicians know it is the right thing to do.

CHAPTER 15

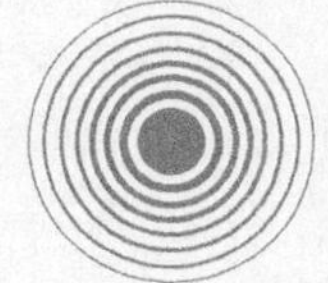

Bridging a Gap: Biomechanics

Biomechanics: the study of mechanical laws and their application to living organisms, especially the human body and its locomotor system.

—Mosby's Medical Dictionary, 8th edition

The medical school training of physicians is limited with respect to some significant pillars for a high quality life—not just nutrition and fitness but human biomechanics as well. *Biomechanics* is a branch of science, which studies the impact of internal and external forces on the human body.[110] Traditional medical students (M.D.s) learn to label and understand the function of the muscles, blood vessels, nerves, bones, and special openings or markings on cadavers in medical school. However, very little is taught regarding how the soft and hard tissues interact with one another in a moving and functional body. Just because physicians can label the designated parts or know their roles in the human body, it does not mean that all physicians understand the various forces acting upon them or among them in space. Some specialties are more in tune with those aspects, but how they approach those understandings can be diverse. I have had multiple experiences that convinced me of the benefits of a biomechanical approach—a valuable tool which has a time and a place, if red flags are not present.

- Prior to medical school, a painful "crick" in my neck noted upon waking was immediately resolved with a gently guided maneuver by a physical therapist.
- During residency training, a patient arrived to the emergency department complaining of pain and the inability to stand up straight after bending over for three hours. After assessing the likely mechanism, palpating, and mobilizing the spine with three maneuvers, the patient was able to stand up much to his surprise. His pain immediately resolved, and he left the emergency department with a smile—*no* medications or prescriptions needed.
- During my private practice, I was able to relieve a patient's chest/rib pain with a simple mobilization technique in the recovery room after the patient had been lying down on his side on a special roll during a long surgery.

Pain can occur from poor positions or movement. If a person assumed a squatting or other awkward position and held it for three hours straight without moving, that person would likely become uncomfortable, feel restless, or experience pain. The person might have difficulty explaining the reason for pain, but would understand the pain would cease once out of the awkward position. Or, consider how different it feels to wear a backpack on one shoulder versus two shoulders for a few hours. It can be the same with biomechanically related *chronic* pain. If the body is in a non-neutral state *for that particular person*, pain can be the result. It may seem hard to pinpoint the cause of pain's arrival, but often there have been repetitive stresses that eventually tip the scale. Insults can add up over time, and the last *minor* insult may have been enough to push the body over the edge, such as a disc herniation while merely picking up a piece of paper. Too much of anything can lend itself to injury or pain. Balanced and varied movement seems to be good for the body.

Most people can understand that walking could be incredibly challenging if part of a leg is missing. Hence, prosthetics or artificial devices were designed to help humans continue to function as close to normal as possible by replacing the missing body part. A more common pain complaint is the "crick" or pain in the neck upon waking. When this occurs, it is highly likely that the pain relates to some poor mechanics during sleep or a recent injury. This type of pain usually resolves within days or weeks if the same sleeping pattern is not repeated or nothing else exacerbates it. Another example is the person doing weight training without the proper understanding of safe lifting techniques or proper body mechanics. If this individual does squats with a weighted bar in an uncontrolled way or in a position that puts unnecessary strain on the back, then injuries can happen. Evidently, poor mechanics can lead to pain.

Elite athletes use biomechanical expert coaches, typically not physicians, to improve performance, minimize injury, and increase efficiency. Poor mechanics can lead to an injury, which can create a chain reaction of other injuries or pain. Elite athletes who master their mechanics with appropriate nervous system training can theoretically avoid unnecessary injury. There is no doubt that many professionals are well-versed in human biomechanics, but most physicians are not experts in this arena unless they specialized in certain areas of medicine or pursue this knowledge on their own.

Unfortunately, if physicians do not have a trained eye to recognize subtleties of the human biomechanics via looking, measuring, or palpating, then the possibility of biomechanical issues related to pain may not even be on their radar. This is like visiting a physician for appendicitis, but the physician was not trained about the possibility of appendicitis. Even in the presence of significant appendicitis symptoms, if the physician was focusing on other diagnoses and no special imaging was available, the chance that appendicitis would be suspected would be very slim.

In the world of *invisible* pain, it is easier to appreciate that an amputee walking with a prosthetic and an altered gait *may* have some back pain. On the other hand, someone who complains of back pain, yet appears to be walking with two good legs with or without a limp, could be questioned about the validity of pain. Plenty of situations exist whereby habits and lifestyle can lead to pain problems. Sitting for long periods of time or working in the garden in a stooped over position can lead to back pain. Staring at the ceiling while painting can lead to neck pain. Pushing weights at a gym in a manner that does not keep the joints in alignment could create wrist pain. Holding a toddler on one hip repeatedly can lead to pain in the lower back or pelvis.

The importance of biomechanics begins early in life, and it depends on the development of the nervous system, which heavily influences the movement of the body. Humans begin the process of moving by crawling. Eventually, with increased strength, balance, and coordination, the body is trained to walk. Over the years, injuries or adaptations may cause mechanical changes. Habits, such as crossing the legs in a certain way or sitting on one foot can affect the balance or alignment of the body's various parts. Men may experience a unique alteration by always putting a full wallet in the same back pocket. Patterns like these do not always lead to pain, but some insidious changes could occur as a response to unbalanced biomechanics.

Although the reliability of palpating or assessing the hips is difficult to verify in studies, hypothetically, small or large shifts in the pelvis can affect everything to which it is connected. Just ask a pregnant woman who has new pain at the pubic symphysis or pubic bone area. Many connections maintain the triangular bone called the sacrum between the two sides of the pelvis. Like a suspension bridge, if one side of the pelvis and all of its attachments is not in balance with the other side, some torque could occur which could affect the sacrum's connections to the pelvis. (see Figure 13) Over time, some rotation of the lumbar spine could occur in response to the pelvis issues, creating changes in areas higher up the spine. Understandably, palpated or visible changes may or may not be related to pain—a similar theme as the potential deception by spine MRIs. It takes highly trained and experienced professionals to assess mechanical subtleties that most physicians do not appreciate, and it can take time to decipher if those observations are relevant to the patient's pain.

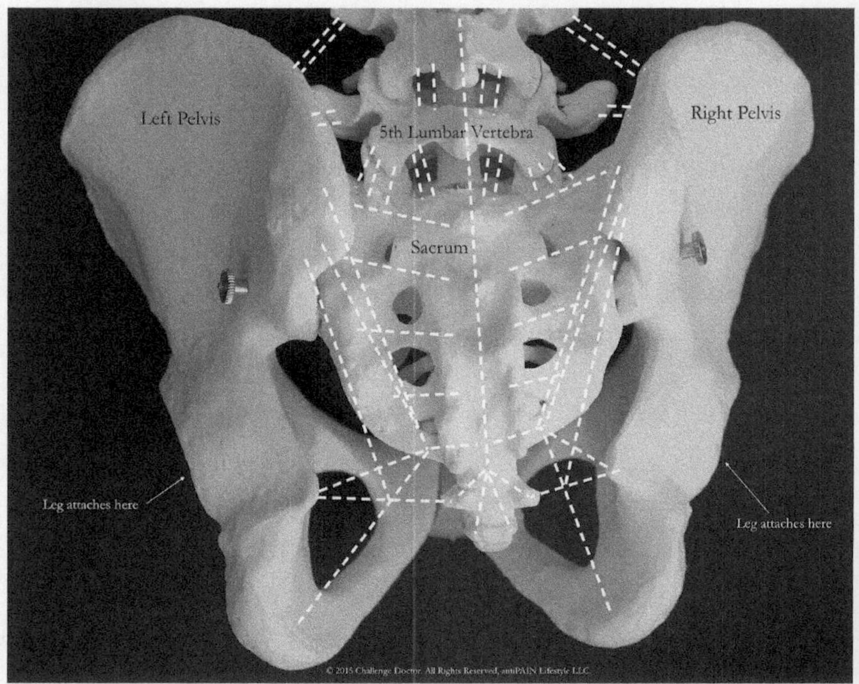

Figure 13: The pelvis does not consist of just bones. There are multiple connections including strong ligaments, depicted by the white dashed lines. There are even more connections beyond these, which keep the upper body from falling down through the pelvis. The ligaments, joints, etc. can withstand great force, including gravity.

As noted before, the body prefers a neutral state. Even though the spine, pelvis or other extremities may be out of alignment, the head, chiefly the eyes, seek to find a level plane. This is why someone with severe scoliosis does not usually turn their head to follow the curve of the spine. The eyes want to be level unless forced not to be. Even in the case of broken vertebra and an extreme hunchback situation, the person's eyes still want to look up and be level with the environment, if possible. As a result, everything between the head and pelvis can change over time depending on the person's lifestyle, conditions, and injuries. These changes may be enough to lead to pain, but not always. Some people with severe scoliosis can be fully functional with no pain. So fixating on an abnormality, especially when there is no pain, may or may not be helpful.[111] Again, it takes an individualized approach by experienced professionals to ascertain the importance of asymmetries.

Many of today's afflictions are attributable to society's repetitive and sedentary lifestyle. Sitting for long commutes and at a desk for almost eight hours a day does not give the body the kind of variety of movement it needs. In expressing pain, the body may be saying, "Get moving or move better." Sitting for long periods causes the front of the body, especially the hip flexors, to become tighter and the back side of the body to become more stretched and over-stressed. If those muscles are never strengthened during activities outside of sitting, then the "glutes" can become weak and lead to less stability. In addition, the back, neck, and shoulders could be at risk for pain.

Active tennis and baseball players can also develop pain through repetitive motion, which can lead to "tennis elbow" or other inflamed tendon injuries (aka tendonitis) of the elbow. Excessive use, increased speed at which the racket is swung or the ball is thrown, or bad mechanics can all contribute to this pain. The pain is in response to stress, injury, or trying to protect the player from further harm.

To avoid pain, there needs to be some level of bracing of the human structure. Similar to a suspension bridge, human stability depends on "geometry, stiffness, balanced cable tensions, and column imperfections."[112] If one side of the bridge has broken cables (*cause*) and leads to crushing or collapsing on the other side of the bridge (*symptom*), then it would make sense to deal with the cause versus the symptom. By dealing with the symptom on one side of the bridge and ignoring the snapped cables on the other side of the bridge, more symptoms can arise. Each human's structure is unique, but *what is done* to help a patient can dictate the biomechanical tolerance later—*what is done* can be influenced in many ways depending on *who* tries to help the patient.[113] In other words, if an initial problem is not addressed appropriately, then a chain reaction of events can occur down the road, which is a common trend in chronic neck or low back pain. Since some biomechanical problems can be progressive, it is helpful to learn techniques from experts to minimize escalation of damage or issues.

Many different health professionals assess biomechanics, yet there is little understanding of it by most physicians. Thus, physicians may be unintentionally misguiding patients when they do not know how to assess or treat biomechanics. If physicians recognize their limitations and the importance of biomechanics, they still may struggle to find an appropriate biomechanics expert for their patients. Each biomechanical practitioner has a unique blending of assessments, skills, and techniques. The most frequently utilized biomechanical experts in mainstream medicine are physical therapists, but they are not all the same nor are they the only people who can assist patients with biomechanics. The concern and risk for the patient is that a biomechanical expert may address the patient's issues inappropriately or overemphasize a diagnosis or a treatment as if muscles and bones are the only issue—yet, other aspects including connective tissue tie into the muscles and bones.

CHAPTER 16

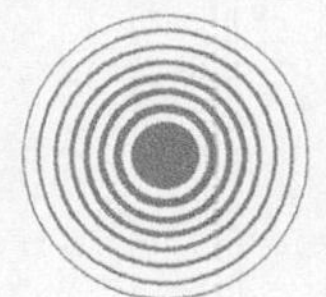

A Missing Link: Connective Tissue

Realize that everything connects to everything else.
—Leonardo da Vinci

No one needs to be told that aging makes the body seem tighter, not looser. In fact, the changes are evident in senior populations as they slow down, take smaller steps, and have a different walking pattern. It is one of those universal experiences of humans; the body becomes less resilient over the years in several ways. This tightness may make its presence known first when getting out of bed. For some reason, it seems more difficult to get up without some stiffness or soreness. This is especially true for people who have *not* been maintaining good health or are carrying extra weight. Usually, after a bit of motion, things "loosen up." There must be something beneficial to motion. Early morning pain is not usually a complaint of most teenagers or young adults. But, for some reason, this complaint becomes more prevalent as we get older.

Humans consist of bones, muscles, ligaments, tendons, a blood vessel system, a nervous system, a lymph system, multiple organs, and more. All these things are encased within the skin, the body's largest organ, which acts as an outer "glove" to keep everything in its place and protected. The human body is well ordered—everything has its place. There is a certain amount of tension keeping the muscles, bones, and internal organs fitting together properly. While skin protects and holds things together externally, *connective tissue*, also called *fascia* (pron. fash-a) keeps everything in its place internally beneath the skin's surface or epidermis. Fascia is the soft tissue component of the connective tissue system that permeates the human body.[114] Connective tissue is a web integrating every aspect of the body starting at skin level, then diving deep into and *within* the muscles and *around* the organs. The human body is not separate parts stuck together. They are intimately interconnected to one another. Connective tissue consists of a variety of elements including *collagen* and *elastin*.

Collagen is a strong protein of many different types but is typically rigid yet bendable. Yet, elastin is elastic and returns to its original length after being stretched or compressed. *As we age, collagen becomes more cross-linked and rigid.* Even the lens inside an eyeball becomes very rigid as we get older which can lead to vision problems, hence cataracts.[115] If there is less or disordered collagen and elastin in the skin, then wrinkles or leathery skin can occur. Again, there is less resilience as we age, whether by years and/or insults.

There are different categories of connective tissue in the human body, but the most abundant is called *areolar or "loose" connective tissue*. Loose connective tissue is comprised of different cell types but the most numerous cells are called *fibroblasts*, which are intimately related to collagen and elastin.

Areolar (loose) connective tissue is everywhere in the body, yet most physicians are never trained on it or on fibroblasts. The lack of appreciation for it starts in the anatomy lab in medical school; skin and loose connective tissue are discarded or get in the way of discovering muscles, bones, or the more "specialized" or dense connective tissues, such as tendons, which connect muscles to bones, or ligaments, which connect bone to bone.[116] It is rare, even in orthopedic surgery books, to mention or elaborate on the less specialized connective tissue. However, many *non-mainstream* health professionals, such as massage therapists, approach a patient's pain problem by working with the loose connective tissue as a basis for treatment.

Fortunately, within the last couple of decades, research has started to reveal fascia's importance and complexity. Helene Langevin, M.D., one of many researchers, is at the forefront of unraveling the dynamic and important nature of connective tissue. She has used advanced technology to observe *fibroblasts*, which play a *major role in synthesizing all of the proteins*, such as collagen, that live within that matrix. Fibroblasts also produce enzymes that can degrade proteins in response to chronic stresses. This reaction is evident when fibroblasts secrete proteins to pull wound tissue together to close an injury.[117]

Much of Dr. Langevin's research stemmed from an initial study to understand why acupuncture needles would get stuck while rotating the needle in an area without muscle. In her work she realized that most acupuncture practitioners were rotating the needle and leaving it in place for thirty minutes, but the needle would *not* unwind right away after the hand was released from the needle. Dr. Langevin noticed that rat fibroblasts were wrapping around the acupuncture needle "like spaghetti winding around a fork."[118] The same phenomenon was viewed under ultrasound in living tissue.[119] The mere stretching of those tissues or fibroblasts initiates a sort of signaling or response to other nearby cells or tissues to respond to the new position. **Connective tissue appears to be self-regulating or changeable, much like the nervous system is changeable**. If this idea is expanded to the whole body, it is easier to understand the implications of certain human postures or patterns and how those could result in connective tissue issues.

This is, in fact, what Dr. Langevin's research suggests. Her human studies using ultrasound revealed a tendency for connective tissue surrounding back muscles to be thicker in people with chronic low back pain.[120] In the lower back, there are alternating layers of dense and loose connective tissue, which seem to allow easy sliding or gliding of tissues over one another, but *those with low back pain seem to have decreased gliding motion.*[121] This decreased gliding motion could be related to fibrosis or thickening of the tissues. Pain signals from this restricted connective tissue could result.

In 2008, further research documented that nerves within the connective tissue actually do send signals to the spinal cord, perhaps when tightness, inflammation, or too much stretch is detected.[122] The brain receives the signal and the suffering person may interpret the stimuli as pain. Research on connective tissue is ongoing that will likely help mainstream medicine understand what is missing in training, such as diagnosing and working with connective tissue issues and perhaps fibromyalgia in particular.

Tightness can show up anywhere, but a fairly common problem is *frozen shoulder* (aka *adhesive capsulitis*). The bones, ligaments, and muscles that make up the shoulder joint are encased by connective tissue, which tightens and thickens in the case of a frozen shoulder. Initially, there is pain with any movement, which moves into a phase of significant immobility, hence a frozen shoulder. There may be less pain in this phase but shoulder function is poor. The condition may resolve over months or years with or without the help of stretching, injections, manipulation under anesthesia, or surgery. In fact, if interventions are approached too soon, the pain and condition can be exacerbated. It seems to occur more frequently in females older than 40 years old, who have had a recent injury or surgery. Because it is more common in women, the debate is ongoing as to whether certain sex hormones significantly affect connective tissue. Some people seem to be more predisposed to this condition than others, including those with other systemic illnesses such as diabetes or other states of poor health. More research is needed to understand the potential roles of hormones and the immune system on the connective tissue. Or perhaps there is something inherently dysfunctional within the nervous system in this frustrating, yet typically self-resolving condition.

A relatively rare condition called *scleroderma* is an exaggerated form of tight or fibrotic tissue. Scleroderma can affect multiple systems but it can affect the skin, which is more apparent to observers. It is not contagious nor does it seem to be inherited. An unknown trigger causes a cascade of events that lead to *increased fibroblast activity*. This increased fibroblast activity ultimately produces one of the biggest problems of this disease—*an increased production of collagen, which leads to sclerosis*. This abnormal hardening of body tissue can damage organs, too, not just the skin. Ultimately, connective tissues are no longer normal, which can have a detrimental effect on the patient's health and quality of life.

On the other side of the spectrum, there can be issues with stretchy or loose connective tissue. One out of 5,000 humans are born with a certain variation of *Ehlers-Danlos syndrome*. (see Figure 14) These individuals can have *very loose joints or unusually stretchy skin* among other signs and concerns throughout the body. The pain these patients can experience tend to be related to the excessive motion of their joints, requiring strengthening or other means of stabilization.

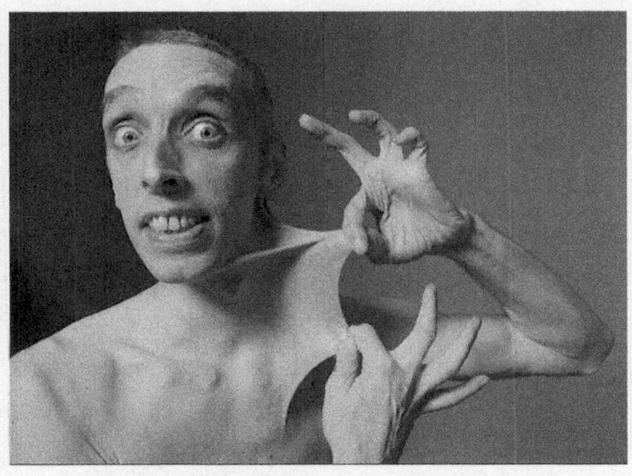

Figure 14: Person well-known for his Ehlers-Danlos syndrome. *Permission obtained from individual.*

While scleroderma and Ehlers-Danlos may not be familiar, most have heard of *plantar fasciitis*, a painful condition of the fascia on the bottom of the foot. I personally experienced this painful condition in my left foot the day after a trail run with brand new shoes. However, the "–itis" insinuates inflammation of the plantar fascia. Inflammation typically involves an area that is red, hot, swollen, and/or painful. The only symptom I had that something was amiss was *painful tightness*. I had the classic symptoms of feeling pain on the underside of my left foot when I first stepped out of bed but it seemed to improve as the day went along. Yet, if I sat for an hour or so at the computer, the pain would return with the next step out of the chair. The more I moved the better it would feel. To give my foot a break, I did more cycling than running to avoid exacerbating the issue. Also, I repeatedly performed massage and pressure point therapy on the painful sites at the heel and arch. Whether it was my training modifications, manual therapy, or just time itself, my pain resolved after six months.

Since the *plantar fascia pain* was not a life-threatening situation and knowing that the body will repair itself with a little facilitation by moving and/or other modalities, I avoided drugs, injections, and surgery again. But most people will not be willing to work through some of this uncomfortable tightness, which seemed to be the biggest problem in my situation. Others would disagree and say that plantar fascia pain is just inflammation and not tightening or thickening of the connective tissue. That may be the case for some people; but, if there is worse foot pain first thing in the morning and it improves during the day, then some of the connective tissue may be very tight or thickened (plantar *fasciosis.*). Interestingly, a study revealed *degeneration* of the plantar fascia with NO inflammatory cells in cases of plantar fascia pain; hence, the validity of steroid injections, which can decrease inflammation and weaken tissues, can be questioned in these cases.[123] Interestingly, platelet-rich plasma, which is derived from the patient's blood, seems to be more effective at healing a variety of injuries with human-derived inflammatory cells and growth factors versus inhibiting inflammation with steroids.[124]

Harnessing the ingenuity of the human body and its brilliant components in areas where it counts shows great promise. Nevertheless, connective tissue problems, whether too tight or too loose, are poorly understood. When issues are difficult to treat, *symptoms* including pain are typically managed in these chronic ailments.

With advances in microscope technology, it is no surprise that additional microscopic aspects of the human body are becoming more appreciated below the skin's surface. As was discussed, there have been studies showing how the rotation of the acupuncture needle creates a stretch in the fibroblasts in the loose connective tissue.[125] Yet, the most amazing part of this is *if the stretch is slow and sustained, the fibroblast is able to communicate with a nearby cell to induce a similar stretch.*[126,127] It appears the connective tissue will eventually respond to what happens to it or within it; thus, it can change with new stimuli and time.

It is quite clear that the body and its connective tissue adapt *slowly* over time. When there are situations of rapid change, there are usually consequences. For instance, a rapid growth spurt or rapid muscle growth in a body builder can create stretch marks. These occur when more stretch is placed on the tissues than they can handle. Pregnant women often lament the stretch marks that develop on their abdomen during stages of rapid fetus growth. Conversely, rapid weight loss in an extremely overweight individual can leave behind a lot of loose, sagging skin that may never retract to its original form. Excessive stretch for long periods of time can make it incredibly difficult for the body to fully recover. In addition, the resilience of the tissues to stretch or shrink tends to decrease as humans age. This resilience could be also affected by genetic susceptibility, personal efforts to optimize health, etc.

On the clinical side, many medical professionals focus on the connective tissue (fascia). There are a variety of treatment approaches; some are very gentle and others more aggressive. Many pain patients seem to benefit from addressing the connective tissue. Some patients respond quickly to certain approaches, while others need help more frequently due to multiple factors including the state of connective tissue tightness, level of physical activity, and genetics. The risk is low in most fascia or connective tissue work unless it is more aggressive, which can lead to bruising or strains.

I have been amazed how some of the simplest and gentlest approaches to issues of painful tightness can create such profound results. I have had bedridden patients devoid of meaningful touch in an inhospitable medical setting receive low back pain relief merely with some sustained inward and downward pressure on their lower back region for merely thirty seconds—no morphine and no ill effects for pain relief, but a grateful and happier patient. Another example is a patient in pain with a severely rotated head and neck (aka *torticollis*) in the emergency department who responded to manual releasing and relaxation of all the tight muscles giving him pain relief and normal positioning.

Connective tissue problems can develop slowly over time based on habits or lifestyle. Since the connective tissue is integrated with the musculoskeletal system, the biomechanics or movement of the body affects that tissue as well. If there is inflammation or restriction in body movement, the connective tissue could become impaired in its function and lead to chronic pain. Interestingly, recent technological advancements and clever research methods have allowed further identification of nerve endings within the loose connective tissue in the backs of *rats*, which could allow unpleasant or noxious stimuli to be relayed to the brain.[128] Further research may lead to a better understanding of the relationship of pain with similar sensory nerves in *human* backs. This promising work from these researchers and others will be instrumental to the understanding of the body—and pain, in particular. Theoretically, delayed back and neck pain from whiplash injuries may be better appreciated with a clearer understanding of the connective tissue's delayed responses, increased reactivity, and association with pain.

As discussed in an earlier chapter, many injections are used to diagnose where the sensory input is coming from in the back, hence blocking signals that the brain could interpret as "pain." One of the injections is the medial branch block, which is done with the assumption that the only innervation of any legitimacy is the facet joint. Yet, the medial branch nerve extends to spinal muscles and other surrounding soft tissues, which contribute to stability and protection of the spine.[129,130] (see Figure 15) The medial branch nerve receives local anesthetic during medial branch blocks but a larger amount of local anesthetic can unintentionally affect other nerves or structures. If the medial branch nerve were not able to transmit sensory input during the block, then it would be reasonable to suspect that the brain is no longer able to perceive connective tissue dysfunction that *could* be causing or contributing to the back pain. Yet, the patient tends to believe that the exam or MRI findings of "arthritis" of the facet joints are the only reason for the injections. The blocks are not as specific as many believe. Although it may help the pain, this block may be misleading physicians and patients as to the true *origin* of the patient's problem. Theoretically, it could be muscles or loose connective tissue and not the bony joint.

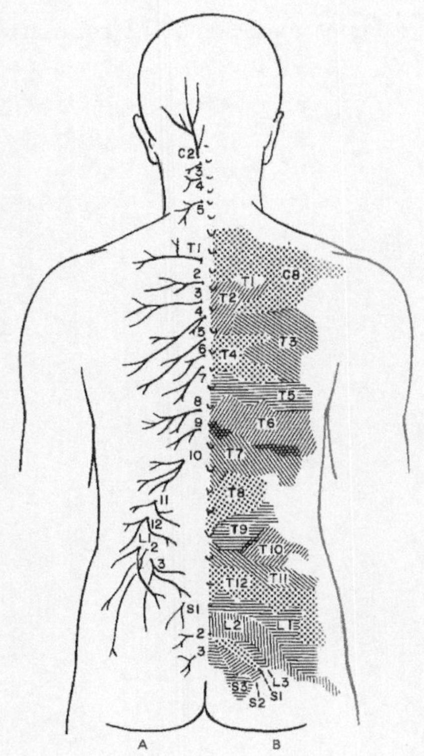

Figure 15: Numbing or destroying medial branch nerves can affect more than just the facet joint. The left side of the back labeled "A" demonstrates the *smaller nerve branches* that come from the spine's bigger nerve roots. The right side of the back labeled "B" shows *areas of skin* that are served by those smaller nerve branches. Although not shown here, deep back muscles are also affected by numbing or burning medial branch nerves. *Permission to use from Wolters Kluwer Health*: Bonica's *The Management of Pain*, 2nd ed., ed. John J. Bonica et al. (Philadelphia: Lea and Febiger, 1990): 140.

It is also presumptuous to believe that surgeries claimed to be successful for "nonspecific" low back pain were actually helping for the presumed diagnosis. Hypothetically, improved movement and less pain could also be related to several other factors including diminished signals sent from the connective tissue stretched by intense surgical retraction. It is hard to control for that factor and difficult to prove.

As mentioned, there are multiple other medical conditions which may or may not be related to connective tissue with varying levels of laxity or tightness. Research suggests special regulation or memory of "loose" connective tissue, but there is still more to understand. Various modalities and treatments target connective tissue or fascia to help with pain and function but the intelligence of this aspect of the human body is just beginning to be understood. Mounting evidence would likely substantiate and reinforce the treatments already offered by so many non-mainstream health professionals who address fascia. Hence, learning and researching are paramount to better understand the connective tissue within the complex human body.

CHAPTER 17

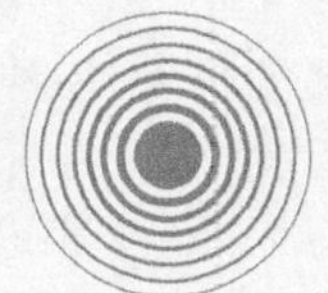

No Brain, No Pain: The Nervous System

If the brain were so simple we could understand it, we would be so simple we couldn't.

—**Lyall Watson**, Author

Despite the importance and interrelationship of connective tissue and biomechanics, the nervous system can override or affect the perception of pain within those areas. In fact, the nervous system is intimately involved with both of them.[131] The brain, spinal cord, and peripheral nerves relate to every aspect of the human body.

What has been so challenging in medicine, pain medicine in particular, is trying to understand the nervous system's influence on pain. With no brain, there is no pain! Sounds ridiculously obvious when stated that way, but pain exists because of the brain. If there is no brain, then you cannot sense pain.

It has been quite common in medicine to direct the treatment of pain strictly to where it "hurts." However, what if someone is hurting somewhere that does not exist? If soldiers lose a leg in battle, most of them experience what is called phantom limb. It is as if they "sense" the leg is still there, the phantom limb, but it does not exist nor can they see it. Yet, many of them experience phantom limb *pain*. The brain is interpreting pain in an area of space previously occupied by the leg, but the limb is gone! If there are no issues with the amputee stump, then training or tricking the brain with a simple tool may help the pain more than a pain pill.

Mirror therapy could do the trick. For a leg amputee, a long mirror is placed between the stump and the intact full leg with the mirror facing the full leg. Then, using the power of imagination, the patient looks at the mirror showing the existing and moving leg and acts as if his amputated leg is still intact. Because of the reflection, the brain perceives the amputated side as being a normal leg with normal movement. After repeated exposure to this mirror therapy, the phantom limb pain can decrease markedly or even disappear. When the neuroscientist, Dr. Vilayanur S. Ramachandran, tried this mirror therapy, there was no evidence this simple, low cost, low risk therapy would work.[132] Yet the benefits were quite impressive. The success of the treatment depends on the type of phantom pain, which means that it will not work for everyone. This therapy is a powerful reminder that our brains are truly adaptive and amazing.

The brain is what notifies the body as to where it hurts, but there are multiple parts or connections within the nervous system to deliver sensory input to the brain. Obviously, vision can send input to the brain that something painful may be *about* to happen and create an *emotional* experience. There are also special sensors or receptors throughout the body that interpret thermal, mechanical, or chemical changes. These perceptions are carried as electrical signals through the nerves to the spinal cord, where there is another station around the spinal cord for interpreting those messages. There are multiple relay stations that have the ability to increase or decrease that pain experience. Those **messages can be modified by signals from the brain as well**.

For example, there is a phenomenon called **wind-up** or **central sensitization** that can occur when pain has been present for an extended period of time.

The message relayed from a painful body part is sent via the spinal cord to the brain. *At the level of the spinal cord* there is an accelerated pathway that develops, which magnifies the pain or increases the sensitivity of the nervous system to the original pain or a new stimulus. In these situations, the pain sufferer can develop *hyperalgesia* or *allodynia,* as mentioned previously.

- **Hyperalgesia** is a condition whereby a patient feels pain *out of proportion* to the physical findings. Perhaps pinching of the skin makes the patient wince or jump in a way that seems excessive in reaction.
    - A specific form of hyperalgesia, *opioid-induced hyperalgesia*, relates to worsening pain despite increasing doses of opioids. In fact, there are multiple reports of patients experiencing less pain as they decrease or wean off their opioids—strange, but true.
- **Allodynia** is pain experienced when a *non*-painful stimulus is elicited. For example, most people would find that a feather stroked on an arm is not painful; however, someone with allodynia in that area of the arm would find it painful. It can be miserable for some patients.

The body has a unique intelligence, which includes the brain, with respect to minimizing pain versus magnifying it. During war, extensive injuries occur in the battlefield, including severed extremities. If near an enemy, the body's intelligence can act accordingly. Under most circumstances, the injury would be so excruciating that the soldier would yell, cry, and focus on the injury. However, with the enemy so near, fear of capture would keep the soldier focused on staying hidden and not the injury. Miraculously, the brain can modify its response to injuries. In the end, the brain is there for survival. If there is danger and a strong will to survive, the brain will influence the situation tremendously.

Yet, there are situations of no pain with serious injuries, and the brain was not triggering any threat. Personal accounts of swimmers in the ocean reveal that an entire arm or leg bitten off quickly by a shark did not hurt. Swimmers may go into shock after realizing what occurred and secondary to blood loss; however, when recalling the incident, they report it just felt like a "pop" but no pain.

The brain can also envision a threat as an adult stares at an intravenous catheter (aka I.V.) needle, ending up in a panic attack before the needle touches the skin. The painful experience manifests itself in the person's mind while merely *anticipating a threat.* This can sometimes be due to previous bad experiences, which the brain has never forgotten. Conversely, a young child could perceive the same needle as *helpful* for the impending cancer treatment and able to watch the placement of the I.V. *without flinching. Anticipatory pain* represents the *emotional* aspect of pain. Yet, there are many other situations whereby one's emotions increase or decrease the nervous system's response to pain.

Being depressed or anxious could make low back pain more painful.[133] When a person is anxious, as in the negative I.V. needle experience above, the mind is fixated on that I.V. being placed in the arm. The emotional distress is typically magnified by waiting for the I.V. to be placed. This delay can increase suffering more than if the person was suddenly stuck with the needle before the person was aware of what happened. This is the reason that distraction such as music or humor helps children and adults in similar situations. If the brain is not sensing threat, then the experience of pain, emotionally and physically, is typically less or minimal. **Yet distraction may not always be a long-term strategy for chronic pain; learning to not be threatened by chronic pain may be more useful for the brain**.

While anxiety can make pain worse, love can have the opposite effect. Preliminary research has been done on early romantic love and the perception of pain. Most people who fall in love have an unbridled passion for the other person, whereby the lovers think about each other all the time and crave to see each other. It sounds a lot like addiction. Research shows that brains with addiction to certain drugs can have a unique brain pattern seen by a functional MRI scan. To see if the pain experienced by people in the early stages of love could be influenced, a research group at Stanford recruited participants who were in a romantic relationship for less than nine months.[134]

Research participants were told to look at pictures of their romantic partner, look at pictures of an equally attractive acquaintance, or perform a word-distraction technique. During each of these tasks, they received a painful heat stimulus. By using functional MRI brain scans, the researchers found that subjects looking at *pictures of their romantic partner decreased their moderate pain experience by 44 percent* and the *distraction method decreased the subject's moderate pain experience by 36 percent.* Interestingly, the pattern that lit up in the brain was different between the former and the latter. In other words, the first was a reward-induced pain relief pathway and the second a distraction-induced pain relief pathway. Most importantly, it is a reminder that rewards and distractions can *decrease* the experience of pain. The opposite is also true. Stress, loneliness, depression, anxiety, or fixating on the pain can *magnify* the experience of pain.[135]

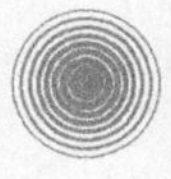

"Stress, loneliness, depression, anxiety, or fixating on the pain can *magnify* the experience of pain."

Fixating on the pain or believing that the pain means something worse is called *catastrophizing.* This is common with depressed or anxious individuals. Multiple behavioral techniques or skills are available to enable patients to down-regulate their own nervous system.[136,137,138] By doing this, patients can decrease the volume of their pain. There are times when simply educating the patient that pain is not due to cancer can calm the nervous system and minimize worry; or learning that the low back is not "fragile" and not going to suddenly fall apart can relieve some anxiety in a highly concerned patient. Simple relaxation techniques that ultimately calm the nervous system allow patients to minimize their pain experience and get back into life.

Everyone begins life with a certain *wiring*—influenced by genetics, the womb environment, and any stresses or trauma experienced along the way. These things can affect reactions to pain. There are "high-strung" people who seem to overreact to every little stress in life. Then, there are those "easygoing" types who don't seem too concerned about anything. If the nervous system were envisioned as a string and stress was like "plucking the string," then an easygoing nervous system would have a lot of slack and would not show much activity when plucking the string. These people seem to have a nervous system that does not highly react to life's stresses. On the other hand, the high-strung nervous system would have no slack in the string and would show a great deal of activity to even the tiniest of flicks or stresses on the string. These individuals may have a more pronounced response to life's stresses, including painful stimuli. An extreme example would be soldiers with post-traumatic stress disorder.[139] Being high-strung is not a life sentence. Neuroplasticity is always present. In other words, the nervous system or pain can be influenced in a positive way by choosing to live life differently.

In pain, neuroplasticity can also work in a negative manner. If people overly fixate on the pain, the areas in the brain light up more intensely compared to those that do not.[140,141] Thus, the brain can change in a negative way. That fixation on the pain known as *catastrophizing* usually leads to pain avoidance behaviors, which usually leads to decreased movement and quality of life.[142,143] The body is meant to move; **fixating on the pain can worsen movement, function, and pain.**[144]

Yet, recognizing that pain is not inherently harmful to the body can improve pain. This is why education is so important for patients. A 2004 Australian study focused on patients with low back pain. A physical therapist or physiotherapist provided education to the patients, which enabled the patients to improve their leg raising ability by 77 percent and bending of the back by 60 percent![145] **By changing the brain's perception or interpretation of the pain with education, the patients were able to improve their function**.[146,147] Research is ongoing throughout the world regarding neuroplasticity and its effects on the body and brain. Understanding how to decrease the volume or intensity of pain can be invaluable.

Overwhelming evidence strongly suggests that education should be part of every pain patient's treatment.[148,149,150] The fact that education can change the body, function, and pain through knowledge, as much as moving the body in the right way can improve pain, is incredibly empowering and useful.[151] Although poorly reimbursed by most insurance plans, time spent educating a patient not only empowers, but also changes a patient's body, function, and pain! Unlike opioids, there is *no* evidence that a patient can *overdose* on too much education—as long as it is *helpful* information. To acquire additional information on pain basics, there are some educational videos and books from leaders in the pain field in the Resources section.

In these last three chapters, I have revealed several incredibly important aspects of the human body that are frequently underappreciated: biomechanics, connective tissue, and the nervous system. Each one of us has a unique level of stability, flexibility, and nervous system control that we can optimize to avoid or minimize pain. The pain journey includes addressing these multiple challenges. Ultimately, the least understood aspect of humans is how *every* system, not just those three, interacts with one another. The **human body and brain is truly *one system* which has an incredibly complex and enormous capability to help people survive and thrive; hence, why I like to refer to that system as the human br-ody™ (brain+body)**. How that "br-ody" is managed is up to the individual and heavily influenced by the assistance chosen to guide the journey.

The next section presents a practical approach to pain management suitable for all chronic pain patients.

PART 3

THE RATIONAL SOLUTION: THE antiPAIN LIFESTYLE

"The antiPAIN Lifestyle is based upon the principles of self-care using healthy challenges and choices which naturally improve quality of life and minimize pain. By honoring a miraculous body and accepting pain's complexity, the medical community would be used as a source of education and guidance to facilitate better function with conservative treatments and occasional bridges (medications, injections, surgeries) that minimize risk and maximize benefit."

CHAPTER 18

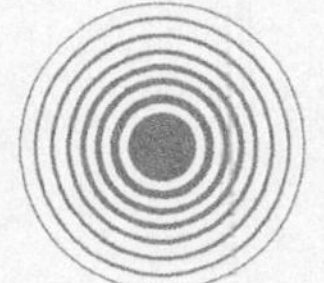

Know Your "Home": Pay Attention to Your Body

Observe, record, tabulate, communicate. Use your five senses. Learn to see, learn to hear, learn to feel, learn to smell, and know that by practice alone you can become expert.

—William Osler

These last few chapters are all about **YOU**. *The writing changes a bit to address* **you** *directly because, in this last section, I share the best ways* **you** *can take care of* **yourself** *and manage or heal* **your** *chronic pain.*

Rule Out Red Flags

The first premise of living an antiPAIN Lifestyle is to rule out red flags. Pain can present itself with a certain intensity, pattern, or character such as aching, dull, throbbing, or sharp. There may also be associated symptoms, which may create fear or concern. If this is the case, then the next call should be to a physician.

It never hurts to revisit what the red flags could be when pain is present, especially since these could indicate something *emergent or urgent*:

- Throwing up blood
- Trouble swallowing
- Rectal bleeding
- Blood in urine
- Loss of strength or feeling in arm(s) or leg(s)
- Loss of control of urinating or defecating
- Unexpected, significant weight loss

Some of the rare conditions that could be associated with pain (especially with the back) include, but are not limited to:

- Cancer
- Infection
- Spinal osteomyelitis
- Spinal fracture
- Cauda equina syndrome
- Dissecting/ruptured aortic aneurysm
- Arachnoiditis

Assuming that you do not have any alarming symptoms and your physician ruled out any urgent or emergent conditions, then what do you do next? You should specifically ask if anything in the history or exam warrants blood tests or imaging. If so, then you should know if there is anything concerning based on all the information. Getting a second opinion is also an option if the physician does not give a thorough explanation despite your requests for more information.

Most of the time, physicians will reassure you that there is a low likelihood of a life-threatening concern present. If no serious concerns exist, then it is always a good idea to proceed with noninvasive approaches before invasive approaches when possible. Your physician may also suggest several things such as patience, lifestyle changes, chiropractic care, physical therapy, or osteopathic manipulative medicine. Patients may not like to be told about habits that should change, but any health advocate should be reminding you of their importance.

Whether you "hear" it or not, your body is always talking to you. Learning to listen to it closely can provide clues as to what is going on. When harmful stimuli trigger nerves to send information toward the brain, a few quick questions can begin the process of understanding the pain experience:

- Was there an obvious injury before the pain started?
- Did the pain seem to creep up mysteriously "overnight?"
- Did you feel pain in the same place before but it went away without treatment?
- Which activities or events occurred the day or days before the pain began?
- Do certain activities make the pain worse or better?
- Are there some bad habits in my life that could be contributing?

It may be helpful to keep a log about your pain to track when it worsens or improves, what helps it or aggravates it, and so on. This log could be invaluable to your health care professional, and it helps you be a partner in solving or helping your pain. There are many online tools and applications that can help you organize your observations. Just remember, due diligence is great but overly fixating on the pain can magnify it.

Below are some signs and symptoms that may be related to the biomechanics, connective tissue, and nervous system:

- Does your morning pain get better as you move around? This could be related to the type of bed or pillows, arthritis, tightness of connective tissues, etc.
- Does the pain get worse throughout the day even if you were fine when you woke up? Something may be stressed or overloaded throughout the day.
- If you previously could cross your legs as demonstrated in the picture, but now only can cross one leg and not the other, this could suggest

pelvic/hip issues that could be related to hip, buttock, or low back pain. (see Figure 16)

- Which position is of the most comfort? Can you turn your head to the right but not the left? If turning the head is restricted on one side but not the other, there are a variety of causes depending on the part of the body and the nature of your issue.
- Is there extreme tightness in tissues, perhaps on one side versus the other?
- Is there a specific movement that reliably reproduces or intensifies your pain?
- Do you tend to be overly anxious and stressed in your life?

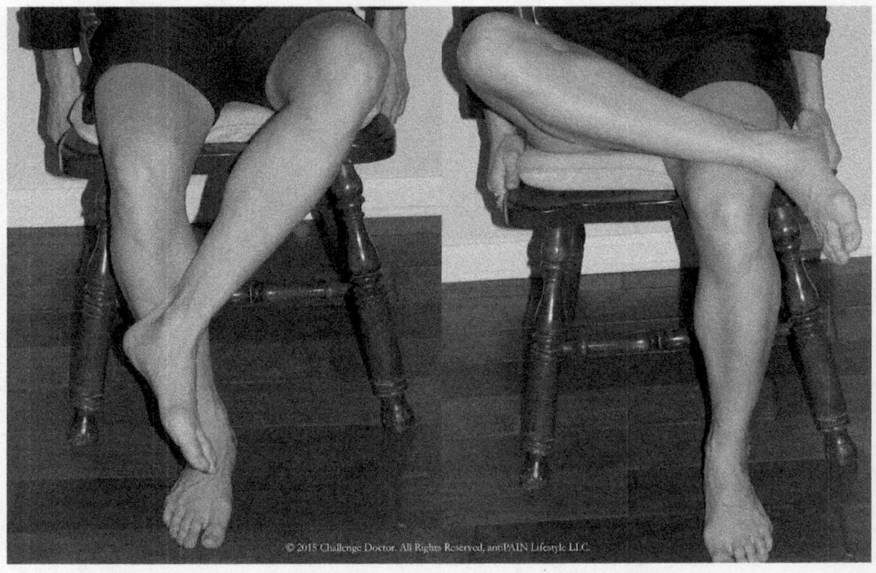

Figure 16: This is a visual comparison of one movement that is different from one side to the other. If asymmetries in range of motion are noted over time and you have pain, then further evaluation may help assess its importance. Warning: The more you pay attention to your body, the more you pick up on or magnify the asymmetries which may actually be normal for you and irrelevant to your pain.

When your pain is not improving despite your efforts or other concerning symptoms have emerged, you should bring this to the attention of your physician or another specialist. Medicine is too complex for patients (or physicians) to make assumptions, especially when physicians cannot see through your body for immediate interpretation. Special imaging, such as an MRI, is merely a snapshot picture of you lying on your back; it may not adequately display the reason for your pain. However, if you have concerning symptoms, then a static or dynamic X-ray or static MRI may reveal some information that is helpful, but be aware of the high incidence of insignificant abnormalities.

Pay attention to what your body is doing or what you are asking your body to do. Remember, **pain is the way your brain protects your body if it is threatened or imbalanced; however, the brain's perception of the pain location may not always be the cause of your pain.** For example, left arm pain can be due to a decreased blood supply to the heart muscle. While your brain is interpreting that you have arm pain, the real cause could be due to heart issues. If you only treat the left arm, then you are ignoring the real cause of your pain. Because left arm pain is a recognized symptom for heart problems, it is unlikely a physician would only treat the arm pain. This is primarily because it can be life-threatening if you have a heart attack. In fact, it would seem ludicrous to *burn* the nerves that supply the heart in place of dealing with the *cause*, which is really the disease of the heart's arteries. I think most people would agree.

However, there are still patients and physicians who may mistake a "healthy" 30-year- old female's arm pain as just "arm pain" when it could actually be a heart problem. This colors the complexity of medicine *and pain medicine in particular*, because what the patient notices as a problem may not be highlighting the actual issue. Just like the collapsing bridge example, the cause can be overlooked when merely focusing on symptoms. Ultimately, if the issue is determined to *not* be life-threatening, then the medical field does not have much urgency to address the *cause* of the pain. More commonly, when the *cause* is NOT known, then symptom-oriented treatments tend to prevail. One of those symptom-oriented approaches is the prescribing of opioids, which, ironically, can lead to respiratory depression and death without ever treating the cause—a true tragedy.

Learn about the "home" or body in which you live. So many people do not understand the most basic aspects of their bodies. I'm not suggesting everyone take an anatomy course, but it is helpful, and could be lifesaving to understand basic bodily functions. This includes knowledge about what each of the "holes" in our bodies does, whether it is to urinate, defecate, sneeze, spit, hear, have sex, etc. I am always amazed to meet patients who lack this rudimentary understanding. Education is paramount to even begin to make sense of your body.

Pain of the spine is a frequent complaint. However, the spine is not just a stack of building blocks, as many patients believe it to be. Anatomy pictures are simplified to label parts such as bones, muscles, and organs. However, everything is brilliantly connected to everything. For instance, your spine is incredibly strong and resilient with extensive tissues reinforcing the vertebral bodies to each other with the disc encased strongly, in most cases. The spinal cord, which lives in a sac of fluid, is behind those vertebral bodies and encased within the rest of the vertebral bony arches. It is rare for someone's spine to simply "fall apart" aside from high speed or extremely heavy load injuries. (see Figure 17) Small changes to your spine do happen over a lifetime; besides, bone is a dynamic and ever-changing component of the body. Most of the time, these changes are due to aging and are irrelevant to any pain complaint. However, as noted in my MRI, these changes are frequently found in spine images of adults—even those not experiencing pain.

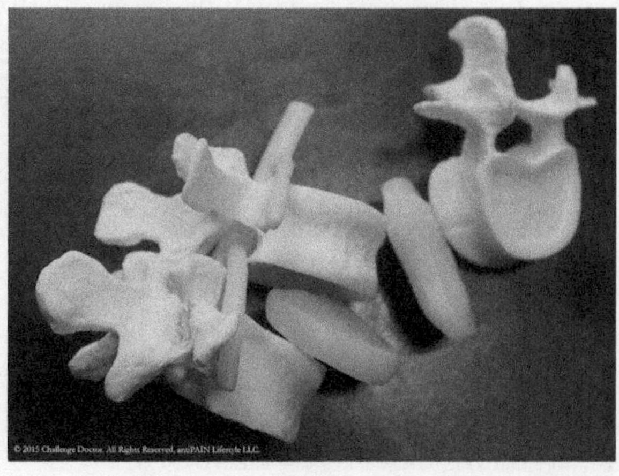

Figure 17: Your spine is not so fragile that it would fall apart like this. Even if the pieces are stacked in this picture, there are many strong connective tissues not shown here that help maintain a strong spine.

If certain areas of your body hurt, you can look up information online from a reliable source to understand that part of your body. However, do not limit your research to just online sources. Knowledgeable health care professionals can help put things into perspective and help you understand if the pain you are feeling is caused by some other area of your body. Your brain tries to make the most sense out of the input it receives, and it can be misleading at times. If you typically avoid moving or doing things you enjoy due to pain, then initially you need to rule out a red flag with your health care professional. **It is important to minimize fear avoidance by obtaining assistance and reassurance with guided therapy to do the things that you initially felt would harm you. Try to understand your body better by researching and asking for a simplified explanation by your health care professional.**

Body awareness is seriously lacking in this country. The less one uses the body, the less the nervous system is trained, which leads to less awareness of the body. You must move and pay attention to your body, because what you notice is part of your story—and your story matters! Your physician can learn from you, to help not only you, but others as well. So, find someone who will listen to what you have observed. It could help the world better understand pain.

CHAPTER 19

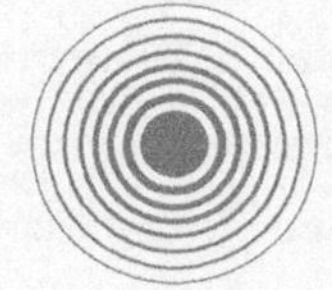

Move, Optimize, and Challenge Whatever You've Got!

Take care of your body. It's the only place you have to live.
—Jim Rohn

Much of what is done in medicine helps facilitate the inherent ingenuity of the human body. Just look at how infertility doctors place a five-day-old fertilized egg into a uterus to allow a baby to develop. Parents don't actually do the replication of cells or do the genetic transcription and splicing to allow an actual human fetus to form. Yet, we do take advantage of great technology to allow a better chance (not a guarantee) for the fetus to survive within the confines of a nature-made uterus. Miraculous. Purely amazing. However, there must be an optimal environment for all of this to occur. Similarly, in life, you must take care of yourself or optimize your body to enable a life with less pain, more function, and more enjoyment as you age.

The aging theory as per the National Institute of Health:

> *No one really knows how and why people change as they get older. Some theories claim that aging is caused by injuries from ultraviolet light over time, wear and tear on the body, or byproducts of metabolism. Other theories view aging as a predetermined process controlled by genes. However, no single process can explain all the changes of aging. Aging is a complex process that varies in how it affects different people and even different organs. Most gerontologists (people who study aging) feel that aging is due to the interaction of many lifelong influences. These influences include heredity, environment, culture, diet, exercise and leisure, past illnesses, and many other factors. Unlike the changes of adolescence, which are predictable to within a few years, each person ages at a unique rate. Some systems begin aging as early as age 30. Other aging processes are not common until much later in life. Although some changes always occur with aging, they occur at different rates and to different extents. There is no way to predict exactly how you will age.*[152,153]

My suggestion is to optimize your own body using common sense with some good science behind it. Be observant, and be honest with yourself. Most problems begin when the issues invisible to the human eye are easy to ignore or deny. For that reason, here are some effective ways to stay out of denial and approach your health from an educated standpoint to minimize pain. See which ones you identify with or which ones may help you the most, *after you have ruled out red flags.*

Listen to Your Body

Being in denial serves no one long-term, especially when you are in pain. Again, listening to your body allows you to keep yourself in check throughout your effort to optimize your body. It is essential. By listening to your body, it is harder to be in denial. Pay attention to how your body reacts to what you do or give it. For instance, some people are more sensitive to certain foods or environments, even if the foods are *natural.* I could tell you to eat almonds—which are considered healthy for people—but if you are allergic and stop breathing after eating them, then it is not a good idea to consume them. Other foods can lead to more subtle symptoms. Make your health and listening to your body a priority. When you are honest with yourself and pay attention to your body's messages, you have a better chance of being healthier and happier. In fact, there are online resources or phone apps that can help you keep track of what you notice.

Accept the Body's Inherent Ingenuity

Your body was extraordinary from the beginning. Do you think about every breath you take? Do you think about killing bacteria that just entered your open wound? Do you command every peristaltic movement that helps your stomach and intestines digest your food? Do you constantly watch your bladder every second to know when to go to the bathroom? As you know, the answers to these questions are usually no. Most of us do not understand, know, or do any of these things consciously for our bodies. It is human to take these and billions of other essential actions for granted.

Our bodies are brilliant systems. I find it fascinating that we get so frustrated with pain to the extent that we think surgery will fix the pain. If we always jump to "cutting out the pain" wherever it may be, then we may be *sorely* disappointed. We now know better that the brain is truly the source of experiencing pain, but where the messages are coming from within the body may or may not be straightforward. Many patients feel as if surgery is the only option when nothing else has worked. If there is no strong data to say that surgery will fix your pain, then it should not be your "go-to" option. Why not provide your body with better choices, habits, and less-invasive options or "bridges" to facilitate what your body is meant to do—move!

Surgery can be extraordinarily helpful or lifesaving in some cases, but it does not renew the body to its *original* condition. Outside of the pain world, surgery is done for a variety of reasons, which may be elective or emergent. For instance, someone may choose plastic surgery to reverse some of the effects of long-term sagging skin. Emergency surgery may be needed to repair a torn or dissected aorta caused by a car accident. Whether for extenuating circumstances or personal choices, the reality is that risk exists with surgery and those risks must be considered.

The focus for pain should be on harnessing the inherent ingenuity of the human body. Destroying or altering the body should be pursued only if convincing data from multiple sources suggests it is necessary or will be helpful for your problem and pain. First and foremost, you must evaluate the big picture and recognize that the body typically heals itself if you are *truly* taking care of it and addressing its needs.

Don't Let Genes Dictate You—Dictate Them!

There always seems to be debate about this, but your gene expression is *not* fixed. Just as it was once believed that the brain was fixed, it was believed that genetics was fixed. Many people still believe it. Humans have a genetic code that is a result of the father's genes and the mother's genes. That same code is in every cell in the body, but the body does not use every part of the code in every part of the body at every moment. Only certain parts of the code are used for certain processes in the body. Would we really make liver cells on our scalp? Would we really make ears on our belly? Sounds silly but there are messages that are sent to our genetic code that let it know what should be made or done next. Moreover, what you *do* every day of your life will also send signals to your genetic code. This is what is called **epigenetics**—an area of study that assesses what turns on or off genes.

Your genetics is a unique reflection of your vulnerability, susceptibility, or tendency toward a certain problem or disease. We all have vulnerabilities to different degrees. Some of us can get away with insulting or neglecting our bodies more than others. **What you decide to do with your body will take you closer to a problem or farther away from it.** There are always rare exceptions—individuals who can get away with more than the average person—such as George Burns living to 100 years old puffing cigars. However, the method of his partial inhaling habit can be debated as well.

Regardless, there are families that tend to live longer, live shorter, or succumb to certain ailments generation to generation. Not surprisingly, the lifestyles tend to be similar when the parents' habits are modeled by offspring. Whether it is smoking cigarettes, dipping tobacco, eating processed foods, infrequent exercise, excessive alcohol, or other lifestyles, there is a tendency to engage in similar patterns. Without realizing that habits may be turning on or off genes, it may be difficult to see the connection to increasing risk for breast cancer, oral cancer, low back pain, a heart attack, or other ailments.[154,155,156] Granted, there are rare genetic flaws that are difficult to change such as a lack of enzymes needed for basic survival. Yet, these enzyme defects are usually discovered at birth or at a younger age and treated accordingly. For others, day after day, year after year, and decade after decade humans are giving their bodies signals, which are molding their genetic code in a certain direction. You have the power to guide your genetics to a certain extent in a better way. Don't let your genes be the *only* thing working for or against you! Your *behaviors* can dictate better gene expression![157] Give your genes better signals with better habits, such as exercise!

Move and Exercise

Moving is essential to health and lends itself to a more efficient body! You cannot cheat this reality. In fact, *sitting has been equated to smoking* with respect to its negative health consequences. Living a sedentary lifestyle can shorten your life. It also pretty much guarantees a lower quality of life in your later years, if not sooner. Sitting or being sedentary, however, is precisely what *most* people in developed countries do. If you remember the negative effects of being bedridden[158], walking is a great solution to avoid those multiple unhealthy effects. Not only is moving important, but moving *well* also helps prevent other issues.

When you move well, you have ideal flexibility, strength, body mechanics, and cardiovascular health. This can lead to a better mind, body, and spirit and often less pain throughout life. If you are too stiff, too weak, too asymmetric, or too winded, then you are heading down a less than optimal path of potential dependence on others and potentially more pain in your life. Recall that biomechanics, connective tissue, the nervous system, and every other system are all responding to the stimuli that you give them. Small to moderate efforts of exercise over the long haul will keep sending the signals to your body and your genes to stay more functional.

If you limit your range of motion or activity as you get older, then do not be surprised if you "cannot go there" later in life—the connective tissue, muscles, bones, nervous system, etc. can only adapt to the challenges or

input it receives. Many older adults who limited their activity to just sitting and minimal ambulation throughout most of their life tend to find their range of motion of youth is severely compromised, which could lead to decreased function or pain. "Keeping it there" is a better idea than struggling to "get it back there." Exercising almost every day even if briefly with an occasional *full* range of motion can help you.

You can build bone density with exercise. A lack of exercise can lead to bone loss and increased calcium loss, leading to other potential problems. With sustained activity, you increase your natural painkillers called *enkephalins* and *endorphins*. Ever heard of a "runner's high?" Runners are less sensitive to pain, more fit, and receive an antidepressant effect from the activity. For those who rarely move or exercise, they will have more tension in their muscles and a higher sensitivity to pain.[159]

A recent study evaluated the relationship between aerobic training and pain tolerance. Healthy individuals who were instructed to cycle for 30 minutes three times a week over six weeks were compared to those who were told *not* to cycle. They applied painful stimuli via strong pressure devices. Both groups recognized the same level of pain, but *the aerobic group was able to tolerate more pressure*. This is another example of how a physical activity can have psychological implications to help a patient reduce or manage pain.[160]

Even if you are not a runner or cyclist, walking activates and, at the very least, counteracts the deconditioning that occurs with inactivity. Always try to gain momentum with activity. *Just moving a little will give more energy for your mind and body*. If you sit around for hours at a time, it is easier to remain lazy. It is important to make your body feel more energy. Energy breeds energy. Moving allows you to increase the energy in your body and helps you feel better while potentially decreasing pain. "No pain, no gain" may not be the best phrase to use when you are in pain, but *if there is no effort, then there is no gain*. In other words, some discomfort or mild pain must be overcome to avoid the occurrence of greater pain later. Remember those returning astronauts who were weaker upon returning to Earth. They had to overcome the pain of walking on Earth again by enduring sore muscles or joints as their bodies re-acclimated to gravity. If they had not been willing to work through that pain, they would have avoided walking altogether. Mild pain and achy muscles are normal when encountering increased or new activity. However, pushing excessively when there is excruciating pain is not the signal you want to reinforce or replicate in a nervous system that is already sensitive and needs to be calmed down.

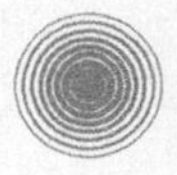

"If there is no effort, then there is no gain."

The question about exercise is how much effort is appropriate for *you*? The focus should be on what you *can* do, not what you can't do. Moving is key and if it is a struggle, then you may need someone to help you. That guidance can help but personal effort is necessary; in fact, **moving activates a cascade of numerous and remarkable health benefits on the inside that someone cannot activate or orchestrate for you from the outside**. Moreover, moving is not like an antibiotic to treat an infection. You don't move as a one-time treatment. You must continue to do this for yourself on a daily basis, which leads to the importance of *adaptation*.

Understand that Adaptation Works Both Ways

Have you heard adults brag about their impressive athletic days in college? Just because they were elite athletes *then*, does not mean they can perform the same way *today* if they have done nothing since then to maintain that same level of fitness. Like teeth altered over time by braces, adaptation of the human body and mind is relatively slow. Nevertheless, months and years do add up, either in a positive or negative direction.

Where does someone start and how much is enough? You should always consider what your fitness level is today. If you have done nothing but sit, drive, and take the elevator, then jumping into an advanced group fitness class with quick movements or other intense workout would likely result in injury, or, at the very least, disappointment when you can't keep up. Some people can get away with pushing aggressively right away without any problems, but often injuries occur because the body has not been prepared for that movement or its intensity. Recall how the body, including connective tissue, adapts slowly over time.

This goes for elite athletes, too, who are only accustomed to cycling, for instance. If you suddenly make them play soccer or tennis, they may struggle because they are not conditioned for that sport and they are more likely to get hurt. You must be gentle with yourself when starting something new; otherwise, the injury turns out to be a negative association with exercise, which leads to disappointment, depression, or just downright delay toward being more active. It's not that your body got "old." Your body got out of shape or became imbalanced. Yes, human bodies tend to become less resilient as they age, but humans are capable of so much more than they realize.

You should be honest with where you have been over the last few weeks, months, years, or decades. Take inventory and start with baby steps. **Seriously, walking daily can change people's lives, physically and mentally.**[161] It may be uncomfortable to just get out of bed, least of all walking. When you get your body going, you do better in the long run. The old philosophy in medicine was bed rest, but now bed rest proves to be counterproductive. The irony of this old passive approach is similar to how the current passive approach of opioids has backfired. **The passive approaches to pain, avoiding pain by not moving or covering it up with opioids, do not serve the population well as a whole.**

If you are in pain while walking and perhaps during weight training, maybe there should be a re-evaluation of how you are living your life or doing your workouts. Are there poor adaptations that may be contributing to your pain? Unfortunately, deconditioning can lessen body awareness, which increases the risk of poor body mechanics. Those poor mechanics can lead to more dysfunctional adaptations. Issues are not always obvious if you are not aware of what to assess. The cause and effect is more obvious if someone breaks an arm. But, more times than not, subtle situations can lead to pain.

What if someone is doing a chest press exercise and his or her wrist begins to hurt that day or the next? There is a possibility that he or she is pushing more weight than the wrist joints can tolerate at that time. Or perhaps the wrists and hands are not positioned in line with the arm to fully support the weight. Your wrist is supported by everything around it, just as the knees are subject to pain if the areas or muscles near them cannot tolerate the stressor. If you don't know how to answer these questions, then find someone who has more expertise than you do in biomechanics. Various manual and movement therapists can help you assess whether your body has adapted improperly or needs better guidance. However, some causes of pain can be insidious making it difficult to trace the pain to a cause. Moreover, the "plasticity" or adaptability of the body is not always explained with imaging or the perceived site of pain.

Appreciate the Insidiousness of Habits

Our daily habits mold our bodies and minds, and it can be difficult to visualize the small changes that occur over time. For example, wearing four-inch heels can lead to foot or low back pain eventually in many individuals.

When humans do not know or deny the habits that may be contributing to their pain and suffering, it is easier to blame genetics or other outside forces. It seems less relevant to do something about it; rather, it is more commonplace to pursue medications or other passive interventions. If we only had some extrasensory perception to truly feel or see the day-to-day changes that occur, then denial would be less commonplace. We are better at seeing the more obvious changes. Why do you think it is easier for us to be impressed by the "before" and "after" pictures of people who have lost a significant amount of weight? It is quite drastic and our brains are easily sold that the person's efforts were worth it. However, the changes from day four to day five were just as important; yet, it does not appear to be a worthwhile change to the naked eye.

What about pain? How can we know that what we are told to do will really help? There is rarely a 100 percent guarantee, but there are some good habits that help us feel better regardless of pain. Fortunately, huge efforts are not always necessary to acquire success or improvement in your health. You must remember that small choices when added up can make a difference. For instance, small deposits of money in your savings or investment account can accrue to $100,000 or more over time. It may not seem possible, but with a little belief in yourself and in the process, you could reach that goal. It takes consistent small efforts and not a one-time effort! If you are creating new habits, then *repetition* will help ingrain those patterns in your brain. That is neuroplasticity at work.

How about another example? Would it make sense to tell your child "I love you" multiple times on one day when they are a toddler or only hugging them all day on one day and never again? Humans intuitively know that love must be demonstrated on a daily basis for it to have a lasting effect. Huge one-time efforts do not. Perhaps you don't want to brush or floss your teeth every day. Why not just brush your teeth once a year but all day? Probably not the smartest idea if you are eating refined sugar and want to avoid cavities. Still not convinced? How about just watering your plant with all the water it needs for the year in one day and forget the remaining 364 days? That plant is alive and needs tending to day in and day out. One day missed here or there is not too consequential, but 364 days of neglect can be tragic to plants—and to humans.

Staying on track all the time would be great but humans can falter; there will be times that you get off course. *Just let the deviations be an occasional turbulence in life.* You don't want those deviations to turn into a new lifestyle, which leads to more ingrained negative patterns, which require more effort to change. Be kind to yourself and talk in a positive way that reminds you that you just got off track *temporarily*. Just jump back into that healthier lifestyle. No one can *do* it but you, but if you need help, then find a trusted friend or professional. As in anything in life, there is no faster way to succeed at any challenge than to find an expert willing to help.

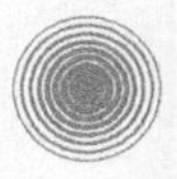

"Your personal lifestyle or collection of healthy habits, *not outside forces or physicians*, will dictate the best health for you in the majority of cases."

Starting new habits is like blowing into a deflated balloon. There is always that initial resistance, but once you get it going, it gets easier as you go. If you fall off the wagon, then you know that there will be that initial resistance at the start. However, you can do it again. Build that brain "muscle" and get it accustomed to *challenge*. You *can* change for the better.

Remember, your personal lifestyle or collection of healthy habits, *not outside forces or physicians*, will dictate the best health for you in the majority of cases. Creating new habits is worth it. Each daily practice forces your body to adapt and respond. To get results in anything in life, you must *act* on knowledge. You just need to believe in yourself and in the process.

Have Faith in the Process—Believe in Yourself!

Have faith in the process of improving your pain, especially if you do not have faith in yourself yet. Sometimes we just need reminders or a different perspective to realize the value of what needs to be done. Whether you need to become more active, do stretches, improve your strength, or lose weight, having others explain its importance can help you build belief. It is human to get comfortable or complacent, but you will reap benefits by paying attention to the smallest changes you experience when putting forth positive efforts over time. Despite setbacks, there are usually clues that good things are happening. *By having faith in the process, you can build belief in yourself as you make progress.* Trust that those small efforts will lead to big changes.

Avoid Dangerous Extremes

Sometimes when you make different or new choices, you may become overzealous and "gung ho" about a new habit. Be cautious of addictions or extreme patterns in life as they have unintended repercussions. Too much of anything, be it exercise, alcohol, shopping, eating, or risky pain medications may feel emotionally and physically great initially. Over time, however, these extreme habits exact a toll and cause unintended consequences. You may be able to get away with extremes from time to time but at some point they will catch up with you.

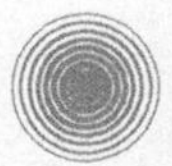

"You must avoid the extremes of doing nothing or doing too much to keep your pain manageable."

If you want to minimize pain in your life, then you must be aware of other choices that could be extreme for your body. If you pay attention to your body, then you know what it is accustomed to doing. Choosing to run a mile or a marathon if you can barely walk a block is too extreme for your body to manage without some significant suffering. A more practical approach is to make choices that allow you to make incremental improvements from your current state of health and fitness. On the other end, allowing yourself to become deconditioned in order to avoid pain is not a wise long-term plan for a better quality of life. You must avoid the extremes of doing nothing or doing too much to keep your pain manageable.

Embrace Variety—Break Physical Patterns

If you leaned over in the garden for two hours straight, do you think your back would be bothering you? Probably. It is likely not natural or neutral for you. However, if you alternated weed pulling, raking leaves, and shoveling dirt into mini sessions versus doing each one fully, then you are breaking the physical pattern or stress on your body. This is the basis for cross training, a fitness approach designed to build strength and endurance by keeping the body guessing, thereby forcing it to be more efficient at managing different stresses. Doing nothing all the time or restricting your movement in one position is not healthy.

Repetition such as sitting in one position for hours upon hours is detrimental for your body. It is no surprise that many people slowly resemble what they do all the time; flexing forward excessively at an office desk tends to lead to flexed posturing even while standing. Just as your brain is able to change, the rest of your body has plasticity as well. To shape your body better, it needs to move with a balanced and dynamic musculoskeletal system and an effective circulation. Instead of sitting all day, at the top of each hour, stand up and walk around or just stand up and activate your muscles in ways that counteract or oppose your sitting posture. Your muscles, connective tissue, and nervous system will be positively affected with varied movement and full range of motion. *Breaking up physical patterns with movement and variety can be helpful for minimizing pain.*

Add Before Taking Away

Initially *adding* something healthy into your life versus taking away those unhealthy things you enjoy can be psychologically easier than feeling deprived. For instance, if you start giving yourself the sleep you need, then you will feel the energy to walk or have better willpower to add a salad into your meal. Those better choices will begin to build upon one another. Just as the insidiousness of your habits can take you in a negative direction, it can also work in a positive direction. You already know that your brain is *plastic* or adaptable. You have the ability to change your brain in a positive way. *The more you practice adding positives into your life then the next positive choice will seem more natural.* At some point, you will begin to take the negatives out of your life as you build up the positives. This can only help you, whether you have pain or not. Something more important must be present before any of these changes will happen—you must have some reason or motivation.

Find Your Motivation

There must be some understanding of the value or purpose associated with taking care of yourself, whether it is walking, eating healthier, or quitting smoking. You must have a certain level of commitment to continue doing the little things consistently in order to reap the benefits. If you do not have a strong enough reason, new habits rarely stick. Sometimes it takes children to inspire a parent to be more responsible for his or her own health. For some people, pain itself is the motivator. If you need external motivation, then you can ask a friend or someone to hold you accountable with frequent check-ins. For those who can afford it and need it, using technology or paying someone to keep you more accountable is an option. *Find your motivation—it will build more belief in what you are doing.*

Quit Smoking

Although some physicians prescribed smoking for weight loss in the past, this is no longer the case for this toxic habit. In fact, the medical profession knows that smoking tobacco is linked to an increased risk for cataracts, heart disease, *low back pain*, *degenerative disc disease*, poor surgery outcomes, poor oral health, and the list continues.[162,163,164] Tobacco is also known to increase calcium loss. Twin studies show that the *smoker twin* versus the nonsmoker twin had a *40 percent increase risk of bone fracture.*[165] Tobacco companies do not emphasize these risks other than what is mandated by law.

According to a 2012 study of smokers with low back pain or spinal disorders, smokers who quit smoking had significantly less pain than smokers who did not quit during an eight-month treatment period.[166] This is very promising for those who have low back pain and want to quit smoking. By discontinuing tobacco of all forms (including nicotine vapors), back health typically improves. It is unclear why low back pain in former smokers gets better; further research is needed. If you cannot quit on your own, then get help from your physician. It may take more than one attempt, but it is worth it. The contents of a cigarette aside from the nicotine, which can be unbelievably addictive, is the way the companies design them for long-term profit—not to mention, they target teenagers or young adults who have the most *plastic* brains to influence.[167]

Studies also suggest that smokers do not respond as well to opioid medications as do nonsmokers.[168] Quitting smoking, beyond the other health concerns, is necessary for chronic pain improvement or positive pain medicine response in smokers.[169] Smoking is an addiction that may be hard to kick, but you will not miss your pain if you take the plunge and eliminate the tobacco (nicotine) from your body. If you cannot do it alone, then ask for help even if you feel quitting might be impossible. Most physicians expect patients to need help quitting due to the addictive properties in tobacco products. People do it every day and you can, too!

Drink Water

Your body is made of 60 to 70 percent water. You cannot survive without it and you must replenish it to allow your body to function and flush out toxins. Your body depends on water. To have optimal health you must give your body what it needs. Drinking a couple of glasses of water when you wake up is a good start especially since you have been deprived of water during your sleep.

Dehydration is not always obvious like thirst. Here are some other signs and symptoms of poor hydration, although these nonspecific symptoms relate to other issues too:

- Bad breath
- Dry skin
- *Muscle cramps*
- Food cravings, especially sweets
- *Headaches*
- Constipation
- *Heartburn*
- *Joint pain*

- Unexplained tiredness
- Dizziness
- Mental changes
- Abnormally dark yellow urine (although some supplements can cause this)
- Decreased urine output (if no kidney failure)

Still don't think water is important? Losing 15 to 25 percent of your body water can lead to multiple severe symptoms affecting all organs. Lose too much and it can lead to death. There is a reason humans can survive longer without food than without water—water is important! However, drinking *excessive* amounts of water without electrolyte replacement *can also be deadly due to a rapid drop in sodium* (aka *hyponatremia*). This is another example of how the body can adapt to small changes over time versus the sudden stress by excessive or large changes.

Hydrate your body with water. Although it is difficult to find guidelines in water recommendations due to extreme variability in individuals, their medical conditions, and environmental conditions, there are some suggested minimums. In 2004, the Institute of Medicine provided Dietary Reference Intake tables suggesting at least 2.7 liters per day for females older than 19 years old and at least 3.7 liters per day for males over 19 years old.[170] These totals are for fluids found within *solid food and liquids*. On average, about 20 percent of water intake is from solid food, but this is highly variable. Although the guidelines suggest sodas count toward this percentage, definitely avoid sugary sodas since they pack on calories with no nutritional value. I have cared for *extremely unhealthy* patients who drank as many as 12 high-calorie sodas per day but never drank water. This is not a healthy practice.

Pay attention to how you feel just after putting water in your body. Just like a plant will wilt without water, your mind and body will also feel less perky. Drinking water will help hydrate multiple areas of your body, from your skin and connective tissue and hypothetically to your spine or joints. Excessive sweating and hot climates can increase water needs for both genders significantly. Thirst usually kicks in to let you know that you need more water. However, if you have excessive thirst without obvious water loss, such as sweating, then speak with your physician. This could mean other medical issues of concern, such as diabetes. If you are not burdened with kidney disease and not taking supplements that make your urine yellow, then noticing small or moderate amounts of darker yellow urine is usually a sign that you need to drink more water.

Optimize Your Nutrition

Your diet is incredibly important—it fuels your body so it can do everything it needs to do. *Everything you eat becomes embedded within every cell of your body in one way or another*. In developed countries, there is more than enough temptation to eat the unhealthiest foods. None of us need help with doing the unhealthy things. We need more encouragement to eat the things that give us the best energy and less pain. Eating a variety of real or whole foods such as vegetables, fruits, nuts and legumes provides many of the specific nutrients given a lot of hype in the media. Yet, there are ingredients and benefits for eating those healthy foods that probably go beyond what we currently can identify or know.

Organic is ideal to avoid the pesticides and other modifications to the food supply, but you can only do the best you can. You can grow some of your own organic food if you are so inclined. The resources at the back of this book give you a place to start. Protein, calcium, and iron are found in fruits and vegetables, not just dairy and animal meat. Beans and nuts also have fiber, which helps keep blood sugars from spiking in your bloodstream like refined sugars can do. If you are aiming to eat *real food*, then you will *rarely* come across a nutrition label on a *whole food* item, such as bananas or kale. For good reason, nature's products are usually not sold in boxes. Regardless, **adding whole foods *to which you are not allergic* can create a wealth of healthy ingredients for your body to decrease inflammation and possibly your pain.**

There are a number of foods that could increase inflammation in certain individuals. By avoiding some of these foods, you may be able to decrease inflammatory-related pain—or just feel better. *Milk, tomatoes, wheat, and eggs may increase inflammation in your body.*[171] There can be others. Each person is unique and sensitivities can vary. Work with your physician or recommended dietary professional to identify potential food triggers that could affect or worsen your pain.

Cow's milk has long been touted as necessary for humans. The milk processing industry has a strong marketing arm that promotes the need for *humans* to drink the milk of a *cow* to have strong bones. However, milk carries potential health risks including increased risk of cancer, allergies, obesity, heart disease, diabetes, and *osteoporosis*.[172] Most physicians are not aware of some of this information. The Harvard Nurses' Health Study followed over 72,000 women for 18 years. The study found that drinking three glasses of milk every day or a high-calcium diet *did NOT reduce the hip or arm fracture risk* in comparison to the women who drank very little or no milk. Yet, vitamin D intake seems to be associated with reduced fracture risk.[173] That does little to support the milk industry's notion that milk benefits your bones. In fact, the countries that consume the most calcium have *higher* risks of osteoporosis.[174] Go for leafy greens (e.g., kale) and beans (e.g., white beans) instead of cow's milk for calcium.[175,176] But, definitely *address your Vitamin D needs* as mentioned below.

Minimizing the consumption of fake or processed foods can help avert the potential harms imposed by the food industry. Processed foods often contain chemicals and other non-natural ingredients that can harm the human body. This includes *refined sugar*. It is hidden in some of the most unsuspected food items and can go by many different names: corn syrup, dextrose, fructose, etc. Note the grams of sugar in the food product label. To give you some context, four grams of sugar is equal to one teaspoon of refined sugar. That would mean that a 12-ounce regular soda has about 8 teaspoons of sugar! Also, pay attention to the size of the servings or the number of servings in that container or package.

Remember, **refined sugar can lead to inflammation in the body**. With a diet high in sugar, there are increased numbers of *advanced glycation end-products* (AGEs). The AGEs are proteins that are bound to the glucose molecule, which results in damaged, cross-linked proteins. Unfortunately, the body's immune system releases inflammatory messengers to break down those AGEs. The long-term exposure to this low-grade inflammation throughout someone's life *could* lead to inflammatory or degenerative diseases such as arthritis, heart disease, diabetes, and fibromyalgia pain, depending upon the susceptibility of that individual.[177]

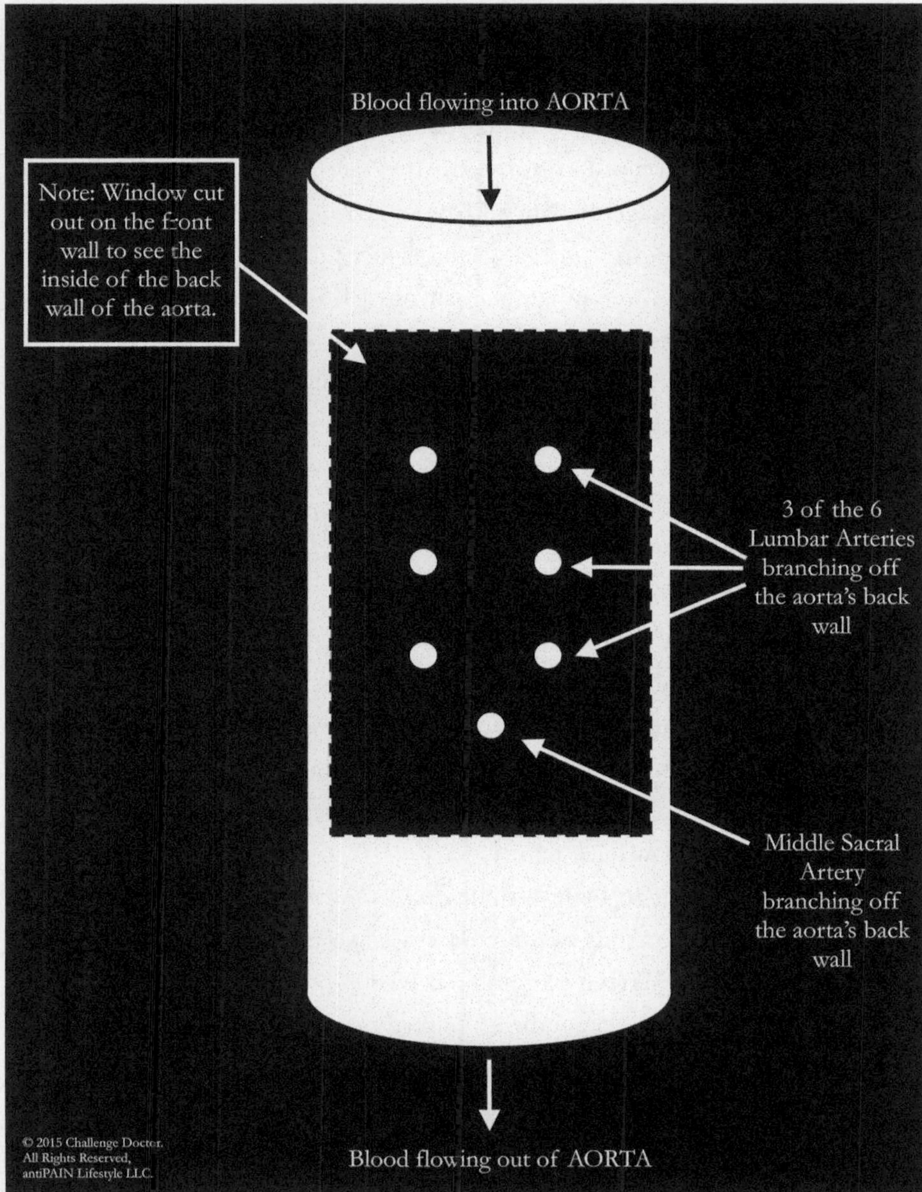

Figure 18: The largest artery, the aorta, runs from the heart and down through the stomach and can be affected by one's diet. Blockages from plaques can occur on the back wall of the aorta leading to less blood supply to the arteries that branch off and supply the spine.

Most people know that fried foods are unhealthy; in fact, they are inflammatory to the body. On the contrary, some healthy oils may help minimize arthritic pain. Avoid trans fats (e.g., partially hydrogenated oils) and minimize omega-6 oils (e.g., corn and cottonseed); they are more inflammatory to the body. Flaxseed and borage oils are anti-inflammatory, omega-3 oils. Although humans need omega-3 and omega-6 fats, evidence suggests you should favor omega-3 fats over the more inflammatory, omega-6 fats. Beans, flaxseeds, and nuts are healthy sources of omega-3 fats.[178]

A less inflammatory or more optimal diet will also enable you to minimize the plaques that could build up in your arteries called *atherosclerosis*. In autopsies, it is not uncommon to see fatty streaks or more extensive buildup of debris on the inner lining of the back of the aorta. The aorta is the large blood vessel that emerges from the heart and travels through the abdomen. There are usually three pairs of openings in the back wall of the aorta which are the starting point of the lumbar arteries. Another opening below those three sets leads to the middle sacral artery. (see Figure 18) In most people, these arteries feed five lumbar vertebral bodies, the intervertebral discs, spinal nerve roots, and the paraspinal muscles that run along the spine. There are studies showing associations between the narrowing or blocking of these arteries with degenerative discs or low back pain.[179]

It may be difficult to believe that *diminished blood supply* could lead to back pain. However, a study conducted years ago unintentionally illustrated this phenomenon.[180] Sixteen patients received *intentional* blockages to their lumbar arteries to manage a condition related to excessive blood supply to the vertebral bones. The most common complication after blocking the lumbar artery was *severe low back pain and spasm* with significant bending of the spine toward the side of the lumbar artery that was blocked. This sounds similar to an acute back pain episode for most people. These symptoms arose immediately or up to three hours after the procedure and took up to 5 to 10 days to resolve. It is not certain if that lack of blood flow improved eventually due to other collateral blood flow from other sources or not. This theory demonstrates how blood flow could contribute to low back pain, especially given the strong link between smoking with *atherosclerosis* or *low back pain*. Many times those two conditions improve with smoking cessation. A win-win.

The lifestyle that lowers *most* people's blood cholesterol consists of more vegetables, mild exercise, avoiding tobacco, and reducing stress.[181] This can help your body clean up the "debris" of the arteries and minimize the blockages that may be associated with degenerative discs or low back pain and heart disease, too. At the very least, those healthy activities can help you also decrease the strain on your back by eliminating excess weight.[182]

There are many natural herbs and other supplements, such as turmeric, that are purported to help with pain but many of the studies have conflicting results. Due to the inability to patent or profit from naturally occurring substances, there is little incentive to do research and very little Food and Drug Administration (FDA) oversight. Here are some supplements that could have a potentially beneficial effect on your pain or nervous system:[183]

- Turmeric is an Indian spice, which contains curcumin, and is touted for numerous health benefits, especially its anti-inflammatory effects. Curcumin appears to help not only with arthritis and neuropathic pain,[184] but recent research on rats suggests that fearful memories may be more difficult to retain with a diet enriched with this compound.[185] Fear avoidance is a big issue for many people with chronic pain.
- Ginger and garlic are common spices purported to have anti-inflammatory effects.
- Capsaicin is an active component of chili peppers and may be helpful for nerve pain, such as pain after *shingles*. Capsaicin can block the ability of the nerve to send pain signals by depleting the chemical messenger called substance P.
- Vitamin B6 is a water-soluble vitamin needed by the body that can increase your pain resistance by its effect on the brain or the nerves themselves. Yet too much supplemental B6 (not in *real food* form) can cause nerve damage.
- Magnesium is an important mineral and responsible for hundreds of processes in the human body, including good nerve and muscle

function. There is moderate evidence that it may be helpful for muscle spasms or cramps.

Supplements, including herbs, are not heavily regulated. Too much of some supplements can be harmful in some cases, and the real and perceived benefits may vary. They can also interact with prescribed medications, or be completely unhelpful. With respect to vitamins and minerals that the body needs, you could be deficient and benefit from additional supplementation based on your medical issues and specific type of pain. **Speak with your physician or appropriate dietary specialist to assess your supplementation needs.** Guidelines are always changing.

The following two vitamins are definitely worth confirming adequate supplementation.

1. **Vitamin D** helps support adequate calcium absorption and retention along with other benefits, including decreased fracture risk, which was supported by the Harvard Nurses' Health Study. Brief, yet frequent exposure to sunlight with or without sunscreen increases Vitamin D levels; yet, excessive sun exposure can be harmful when unprotected.[186] However, if you do not get adequate sunlight or are not sure if your vitamin D levels are adequate, then speak with your primary care physician about your need or dosages for supplementation.
2. **Vitamin B12** (*aka* cobalamin or cyanocobalamin) is essential for a healthy nervous system, which includes the brain. It is not made by plants or animals, but rather by simple bacteria. Since it is found in dirt or other animals' intestines, adequate levels may not be met with dietary consumption if avoiding animal products or practicing modern hygiene. Ideally, to avoid the possible harmful effects of the manufacturing of animal meat products, you can obtain B12 in enriched foods, such as nutritional yeast or other supplementation, which you can discuss with your personal physician or other appropriate dietary specialist.

Before spending a lot of money on supplementation, however, try *real food.* Most of what you need exists in whole foods, with a heavy emphasis on plants. An overwhelming amount of conflicting information exists regarding nutrition, but keeping it simple with *real food* gives you a better chance of getting what your body needs. To be successful, you must make healthy food a priority and be purposeful in which foods you prepare for your next day or week. Otherwise, you can fall into the trap of convenience foods, which are typically not healthy. Of course, the nutrient density or quality of store-bought foods is not always known; consider a farmer's market for less expensive, fresher, and more organic options. If you are not sure how to prepare healthy foods, community or online resources can give you some ideas. See the Resource section at the back of this book.

There is an overabundance of unhealthy foods in our developed country. If you fail to plan your *healthy* food items, then it is easy to fall off the wagon. Start creating the habit of finding your favorite healthy foods. Your palate will begin to enjoy *whole foods* more as you steer away from too much unhealthy food... neuroplasticity is still in effect!

Sleep Well

There are multiple studies suggesting a strong association between non-restorative sleep and widespread pain.[187] It is hard to say if the poor sleep is causing the pain or if the pain is worsening the sleep, but it is known that impaired sleep can exacerbate pain by causing hyperalgesia (*increased sensitivity to painful stimuli*).[188,189] Then, there is opioid use. Opioids decrease the amount of time in deep or restorative sleep.[190] Obstructive sleep apnea, especially if undiagnosed and untreated, can lead to ineffective sleeping as well. You can see how crazy this vicious cycle can be. More pain leads to less sleep but more opioids worsen sleep and sleep apnea. All of that poor sleep can make pain worse.

You definitely want to find ways to get better sleep. Getting exercise can help with better sleep, but you may want to avoid the strenuous exercise right before sleeping. Limiting opioids, alcohol,[191] or caffeine intake can improve sleep as well.

If you are going to try to start good habits, it is always good to start the night before with a great night's sleep. The next day your outlook and energy will give you a powerful mental advantage for tackling the healthier habits upon which you are about to embark to help decrease your pain.

Manage Weight

Do not let your weight get in the way of being mobile and maintaining healthy habits. If your body cannot move because you are deconditioned and too heavy, then you are over-stressing your musculoskeletal system. For many people, their susceptibility to weight gain can lead to health issues, although many thin individuals can be unhealthy on the inside, too.

Why is too much weight important? In data obtained from over *one million* adults collected from 2008 through 2010, there were **substantial pain increases as patients became more obese**, based on BMI (weight in kilograms/height in meters squared). Although *I do not agree with BMI as a perfect indicator* for the health status of humans, these were the findings:

GROUP	BMI	Compared to those with BMI<25
Overweight	25-30	20% more pain
Obese I	30-35	68% more pain
Obese II	35-40	136% more pain
Obese III	>40	254% more pain

By the data above, it would appear that a healthy BMI less than 25 is ideal but once you get above 35 there is a noticeable increase in pain. Yet, the BMI number is a very crude estimate of body fat, which is not always reflective of the fitness or the function of the individual. In fact, if you look at fit New Zealand rugby players, they are considered obese based on BMI numbers. The health of the rugby player is usually better than what their BMI indicates. I would surmise that they "hurt" on a more regular basis than the average American with the number of hits they take during a rugby match without pads or helmets. Regardless of what you do, if you have a **BMI>40**, then you have the potential of **254 percent more pain** than someone with a BMI<25![192]

Remember, weight gain that occurs slowly may not lead to pain for a while. In contrast, if you suddenly put 150 pounds on your back by carrying someone else up a mountain, not only would it be more difficult, but you may feel some aches and pains until you take that person off your back. Your body is telling you that you are going too hard, too fast, or both for it to keep up. For someone who carries that weight internally, there is a tipping point when the body or joints have incurred too much stress over an extended period. It is all too common for a pregnant woman to have back or pelvic pain during her last months of pregnancy; yet, many times it resolves after the baby is born. Or perhaps, a hefty professional football player receives repetitive stresses on the body and joints over many years; his body could end up with cumulative damage and pain. It could have a lasting effect on his joints and function.

Your weight is more important than you think. The heavier you become, the more pain you can have. The worst part about gaining weight is how easy it is to deny the small amounts of weight that increase over time. Before you know it, the weight to take off can seem overwhelming. By applying many of the lifestyle approaches in this chapter, your weight will typically begin to normalize, but you cannot focus on one thing at the exclusion of everything else. Take an honest assessment of your weight and how you function in life. Then find some help or just start with whole foods, water, and increased activity such as daily walking. Your body will adapt and change. *Remember, the effort precedes the visible change*. By being an *active* participant, you can make that change as long as it is consistent with the right habits or signals to convince your body and genes to be healthier.

Avoid Passivity

The world is filled with technology, but it does not exclude the need to take care of your body. Even though society as a whole does not need to work as hard physically or emotionally to survive in life, **we all need reminders to do more than we are doing**. Unfortunately, many times we receive the *wrong* cues for a healthy and happy life. Many of those messages come from social media, including commercials or advertisements. They make strong suggestions or glamorize items or choices that over a lifetime lead to unhealthy bodies and minds. It is inevitable that our environment molds us. Human brains are *plastic*, for better or for worse. The reality is that we all have a choice despite the barrage of influences. None of us needs help with the bad things. More influences that are positive would serve us better. Thus, we can choose to educate ourselves and make more informed decisions.

Not all choices are easy. It is easier to be passive and not take responsibility for your health or happiness. Successful and unsuccessful people all have the same hours in a day; neither really enjoys doing the things it takes to be healthy or successful. Yet, those people who are more successful or in less pain typically decide that doing those things is worth it, despite the sacrifice or effort.

Why do most people choose not to put forth the effort? First and foremost, it is too much work or discomfort, especially if they are already in pain. In developed countries, most of our needs are met with so many more fun things to grab our attention. Yet, you must convince yourself somehow to want or desire the inconveniences such as eating real food or being more active so that you can have the delayed gratification of a better quality of life. Often there are half-hearted attempts by physicians to mention the importance of diet, fitness, strength, flexibility, and lifestyle. This may stem from a physician's lack of education as to its importance, lack of application to the physician's own life, lack of belief that the patient will be inspired to make a change, lack of time, or perhaps financial incentives to *do* something *to* the patient. Yet, when you are in pain, it is more important to focus on doing the healthier things. **Just as someone with a strong predilection for heart disease needs to optimize diet and exercise, pain sufferers must challenge themselves to optimize their lives as well.**

Life is precious and too short. In order to have the quality of life that you are capable of having, you must cherish yourself and do things that lead to a happier and healthier life. I know this sounds idealistic, but **what you should do to make the biggest difference in your own health is to repeat the simple things over and over again**.

Which areas in your life are you following an unhealthy path because of peers or the media? Make a choice to make better decisions and stick to it, despite going astray occasionally. Moreover, if you are not already, surround yourself with positive role models—you will become more like them.

Connect and Love

One word
Frees us all the weight and pain of life:
That word is love.
—**Sophocles** in *Oedipus at Colonus*

Often we do better when we feel heard or are around others who suffer from similar painful afflictions, whether emotional or physical. Finding a support group can be therapeutic or just a great starting point to start adding more healthy activities to your life. There is accountability when you have social support but more importantly, the connection gives people a sense of importance and purpose. However, be wary of negativity and complaining that can become infectious and unhealthy for your mind. Just as a child imitates their parents, we are all vulnerable to different degrees of mirroring one another. Humans can make the mistake of surrounding themselves with people and environments that enable poor habits. When you want to make changes in your life, positivity and healthy competition with yourself or others can give you the nudge you need to do the things that help you with your pain.

Surround yourself with love, support, and healthy environments. It does a brain good and helps improve your pain in the process. Besides, it has been shown that romantic love can decrease moderate pain by at least 40 percent.[193] Astonishingly, one of my prior patients who had received extensive opioids and invasive interventions no longer had pain at his last appointment. When I asked him what helped, my patient replied, "I fell in love." Whether it was love itself or the motivation to get out and move, it is hard to know.

It is ironic that one of the most complex and troubling human experiences, *love*, can help decrease another complex and troubling phenomena, *pain*. As an insightful leader stated, "Love is a lot like pain."[194] Love and pain can be hard to quantify, difficult to prove in studies, overwhelming to the senses, uniquely experienced from person to person, can lead to suffering, affect brain chemistry, and you know it when you see it—or at least we *think* we do. "Obviously they are NOT the same, yet considering their similarities can help us understand pain as more than only a *medical* condition. In reality, pain and love can adversely impact our ability to function and think clearly, and the pain of love-lost is as real as a broken bone."[195]

Do not isolate yourself. Stay connected with others—and not just by Facebook!

Acknowledge Pain—Minimize Distraction

Have you done something that you did not necessarily enjoy, but because you were listening to music or talking to a friend, the time seemed to fly by? Sometimes, you can use distraction during exercise to help motivate you, such as music[196], a willing friend, TV, or using a timer. **Distraction can be a very effective short-term strategy for pain relief, but it may not be a long-term strategy for chronic pain.**

When suffering from chronic pain, the goal is to train your brain to interpret the current situation as less threatening. If there are no red flags, you must be able to *acknowledge your pain* as not damaging and work through it to diminish the pain signal interpreted by the brain. Your brain is trying to protect you from what it *perceives* as a threat. If you ignore chronic pain by distraction, the signal gets louder until you stop due to escalating pain. **When you approach an activity or exercise, you must teach your brain that what you are doing is not harmful**. As you do the activity, you must tell yourself that this will not harm you now or tomorrow. The key to success, however, is moving through the activity at a level where there is only a little to no pain, so as not to overexcite the nervous system. By doing this you can convince your brain that you are fine.

You do not want to pay the price of overdoing it when you have chronic pain, but there must be a constant effort to increase your activity while teaching the nervous system that no danger is present. Hence, distraction may work in the short-term but it does not necessarily have long-term benefits for chronic pain. If you want to train your brain to view your pain as non-threatening, then you must acknowledge the pain as not harmful during activities.

Practice Mindfulness/Meditation

In light of the fast pace and distractions of developed society, it is no surprise that it becomes very easy to move to the next distraction without being fully present in the current moment. This is where mindfulness comes in. *Mindfulness* has become a more commonly used term to emphasize non-judgmental awareness of one's thoughts, feelings, and bodily sensations. If you suffer from anxiety, depression, or pain, mindfulness helps you become aware of the little things within you and around you. It is a way to decrease stress, anxiety, depression, and *pain*. It can also be a good practice to prevent overeating or to improve your sleep.[197] However, there must be a willingness to be comfortable with an idle or more relaxed mind. You must be able to be "in the moment" and accepting of it. It is not always easy for people to calm their mind when they are accustomed to racing thoughts and constant distraction or pain. Yet with practice, *your mind and body can become better at calming your nervous system.*

There is extensive research being done on the effects of mindfulness or meditation on the brain. One particular study compared subjects who meditated 45 minutes daily with those who did not meditate. It showed that parts of the brain associated with attention, perception, and sensory processing were thicker in those who meditated. In addition, the changes were most notable in older subjects, which suggest that meditation might minimize age-related thinning of the brain. The more you meditate, the more certain parts of your brain thicken.[198]

If 45 minutes seems like too much time to meditate, the simple practice of breathing can elicit a more relaxing effect on your sympathetic nervous system or fight-or-flight system. As little as five or ten minutes a day spent doing slow, *deep breathing* can change your perspective, anxiety, and reduce your pain. Some people turn to their *faith* or *religion* to enhance their perspective in life. There is evidence that some people find *binaural beats or tones* to be effective at decreasing stress, anxiety, and chronic pain, including migraines and other headaches.[199,200,201] For others, essential oils or aromatherapy seems to be therapeutic.

Sometimes you may need help in understanding your thought patterns, which may not be serving you. There are extensive online and community resources to assist you with learning and maintaining a mindfulness and/or meditation practice. Changing your perspective and understanding your mind's connection to the body can be a powerful tool to decrease the suffering associated with pain.

Simplify Life, Decrease Stress, and Be Creative

Sometimes part of being mindful is being aware of the life that you have created for yourself, such as your job, friends, and commitments. If life seems too overwhelming, which can seem worse when experiencing pain, then it may be time to evaluate what is important in life, with whom you surround yourself, and how you spend your days.

- Are you ignoring self-care when your health is suffering?
- Are you saying yes to everyone's requests to please them?
- Do you find little time for yourself because too much is scheduled?
- Are you financially strapped but spending more than necessary?

If stress is the norm for you, then it can be easy to underestimate or deny the stress upon which you are under. If you go on vacation for a week and feel the dread of returning to work, then significant work stress may exist for you. For anyone with stress or a perfectionistic tendency, positive reframing, acceptance, and humor can have a powerful effect on dealing with struggles or perceived failures.[202]

Do you recall how interconnected the nervous system is with every aspect of your body? Stress and personality traits can affect your posture or body mechanics, which can put you at risk for further pain.[203] Have you noticed how your life or your pain affects how you carry yourself?

Be honest with yourself. Only *you* know what is making your life more complex; however, at times a good friend or respected leader in the community can help you see what is complicating your life. If you are not content in the life that you have chosen for yourself, then evaluate it. You live in a country of choices. Even patients who have endured catastrophic events choose to overcome or succumb to them. Make choices that simplify your life and decrease stress—it helps your mind and body. It can help lessen your pain, emotionally and physically.

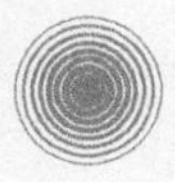

"Find a creative way to design a healthier or antiPAIN Lifestyle!"

We all have the same time in a day; thus, creativity is important if stuck with tight schedules. All of us must re-evaluate our lives and decide where to put our time. Sometimes we must reinvent our careers or lives based on multiple factors, especially if it is contributing to pain. There are very few situations when your employer will put your health before any of their business objectives. Thus, **you** must make your health a priority or it could suffer. Aside from your own family and personal obligations, there is also social media competing for your attention. To find time for your health, you may need to delegate certain tasks, say no to requests that are not in your best interest, exercise with your children, stretch at work, or whatever works for your particular situation. **Get creative, but above all, demand sanity for your life and your health.**

Find Passion, Have Fun, Laugh, and Smile!

We shall never know all the good that a simple smile can do.
—Mother Teresa

By becoming more mindful and simplifying your life, it becomes important to reflect on the activities that you enjoy or could enjoy. Being passionate about something you do can help you enjoy life *despite pain.* It may take some effort or discovery, especially if you are like many Americans who have gone from *structured* schooling to a *structured* job that supports a *structured* or routine family life. Yes, among that structure can be some inherent chaos or monotony; however, many adult Americans do a poor job with structuring FUN after getting into a routine.

It can be challenging to find the time but if you do not make the time, then fun is unlikely to happen. It is in finding passion and having fun that can lead to less pain and more laughter. **Genuine laughter has been shown in studies to increase pain tolerance and improve quality of life.** Laughing can also affect the brain's chemistry—there is an increase in the "feel good" chemicals such as dopamine and decrease in the stress hormones such as cortisol.[204]

If you cannot muster up enough passion and fun with your pain right now, then most of us have the capacity to smile. Smiling can help your pain in ways that many do not realize. Some studies suggest that fake smiles can still affect the brain. So fake a smile until it is real. When it is real, then your smile will engage the eye muscles and have more impact on how you feel. Even if you desperately want people to know you are in pain with your frown, try smiling instead. As Mother Teresa suggested, it's a *gift* to someone else who may be suffering, too. And that should make you feel good.[205]

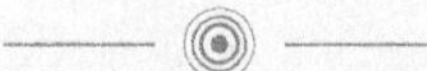

Especially in developed countries, one's happiness and health are derived from more effectively navigating this world with multiple skills that help us avoid the numerous enticements, challenges, and potential addictions. Whether you realize it or not, each of the above topics has relevance to your life and your pain. Layering each of these compensations in a positive manner can act in a synergistic way; hence, you can improve your situation more profoundly by addressing multiple issues versus only one. Attacking one at a time may be all you can do, but over time you can layer those efforts and create a more significant impact on your health and pain. To make it easier, link a new behavior with an already established daily or frequent activity to help your brain transform that new behavior into a habit more quickly. Sometimes you can accomplish these challenges on your own, but sometimes you may need friends, family, or experts to guide you in the right direction. Besides, *appropriate* experts can save you time by avoiding the frequent pitfalls or mistakes made by less-experienced individuals.

Never let getting help deter you from taking care of your "home" or body in which you live. It is always acceptable to ask for help. Of course, some well-intentioned health care professionals, friends, or family may make unhealthy suggestions, such as opioids or other invasive options as the first choice. You must realize where those decisions can end up taking you. Be careful what you demand—you will likely get it—whether you need it or not. Those choices are yours, but if your pain is interfering with your life, then discovering other options is essential unless you are one of the lucky few whose chronic pain self-resolves quickly. The following section includes options that many people in pain have found helpful. It may start with researching various resources in your area, online, or through your physician.

As a reminder, challenging yourself to change your habits will allow you to see change. You must never forget that the effort must be continual and it will always precede the tangible change. Be patient. You do not need to be perfect in every aspect of your life, but you must become better at more areas of your life more often than not. Find your health challenge—it is not just in the knowing, but also in the doing. Your pain experience has a better chance to improve when you take charge of the habits that decrease your pain. You be the judge.

antiPAIN Lifestyle Reminders	Check (✓) areas needing most improvement
Listen to Your Body	
Accept the Body's Inherent Ingenuity	
Don't Let Genes Dictate You—Dictate Them!	
Move and Exercise	
Understand that Adaptation Works Both Ways	
Appreciate the Insidiousness of Habits	
Have Faith in the Process—Believe in Yourself!	
Avoid Dangerous Extremes	
Embrace Variety—Break Physical Patterns	
Add Before Taking Away	
Find Your Motivation	
Quit Smoking	
Drink Water	
Optimize Your Nutrition	
Sleep Well	
Manage Weight	
Avoid Passivity	
Connect and Love	
Acknowledge Pain—Minimize Distraction	
Practice Mindfulness/Meditation	
Simplify Life, Decrease Stress, and Be Creative	
Find Passion, Have Fun, Laugh, and Smile!	

CHAPTER 20

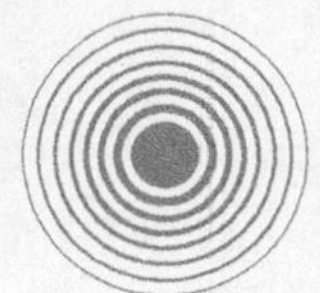

Do-It-Yourself Pain Management?

The aim of medicine is to prevent disease and prolong life, the ideal of medicine is to eliminate the need of a physician.

—William J. Mayo, M.D.

Sometimes you may not be sure of the pain's origin, but let's assume you have received a medical opinion that there is no evidence of serious disease. If you choose to work on your body, then multiple exercises or activities are available that will have an impact on the biomechanics, connective tissue, and nervous system. They can potentially help your pain. Learning physical ways to prevent or relieve intermittent or constant pain are just as important as participating in social activities that keep the mind active.

We all know that doing nothing and being lazy is not good for your body. So if you choose an activity to do in the comfort of your own home, at a studio, or at a gym, then find a resource or an instructor who recognizes that beginners must *start low and go slowly*. Your body adapts slowly to everything you do. You may feel good enough to do things, but starting slowly and advancing in small increments can help you avoid injury. It is counterproductive to associate *extreme* pain with effort. You can hurt yourself even in yoga. **Slow is better than fast, especially when you are just starting out or in pain**. Every aspect of your body must adapt to new or increased activity. Using this wisdom, you will be less likely to scare yourself away from healthy behaviors due to injuries or excruciating pain!

Here is a list of healthy *body and mind* activities for individual or class settings that have minimal to moderate evidence for improving or preventing pain:

- Yoga, in its many forms[206,207]
- Tai Chi, in its many forms
- Qigong
- Pilates
- Alexander Technique: originated around 1910s[208]
- Feldenkrais® Method: originated around 1940s
- Gyrotonic®/The Gyrokinesis® Method
- Mitzvah Technique: modification of Alexander & Feldenkrais®
- Dance Therapy[209]
- Hanna/Clinical Somatic Education

By no means is this list exhaustive. See the Resources section at the end of this book for some online sources of information. There are many other forms of body movement and awareness methods. Yet, **there is an obvious common theme to all of the above—they make you "move" in more ways than the typical American "couch potato."** You may also develop valuable friendships or a sense of belonging. *Movement is essential to good physical and mental health.* The techniques and incorporation of slow and deep breathing patterns can ultimately calm your nervous system. If you commit to the effort, then these activities can help you become more aware and mindful of your mind and body, thereby decreasing the pain signal. What is learned in these classes can be carried over to personal use at home, if you choose.

Sometimes what you do for yourself may not seem to be enough to decrease or eliminate pain. Yet, you must ask yourself if each effort showed even a small improvement. You must notice each small positive change so you can continue to do the things that are moving you toward balance and away from pain. You are human; you will have good and bad days but the overall progression should average out in a positive direction.

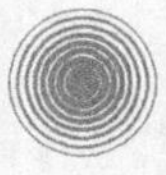

"You must notice each small positive change so you can continue to do the things that are moving you toward balance and away from pain."

It may take time for results that are more impressive. Your progress depends on such things as how long your chronic pain has been present, your age, your effort, and other factors. However, that's OK. Like losing weight, slow and steady in the right direction is more sustainable, and it is still progress. I assume your goal is to reverse or decrease pain eventually. Overnight success is not always the case for everyone. If your do-it-yourself efforts have not been effective in a consistently positive way, then the next chapter addresses options for assistants who can facilitate a more harmonious body and mind with less pain.

CHAPTER 21

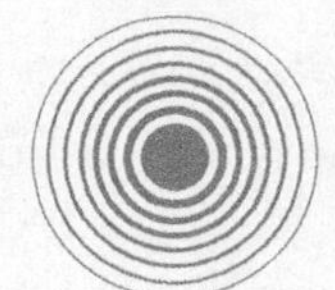

Who are Your Body and Brain Assistants?

...the assistance provided by health professionals is largely a matter of guiding, coaching, and facilitating self-management.

—**Institute of Medicine**, *Relieving Pain in America*

One of the toughest responsibilities that I have is trying to help patients see their chronic pain from a different perspective. For example, just as your ideal nutrition or optimal weight is not going to come solely from taking a pill, the same applies to chronic pain, such as back pain. Pills and injections do not teach life skills; thus, they should only be used to help facilitate other therapies or better function. A random epidural steroid injection or narcotic pill is not necessarily going to fix all of the potential contributors of pain. In a few instances of injections, the pain may improve indefinitely, but it could have been a placebo effect, whereby the patient is pleased to have something done or believes in it. Many times it is assumed that the treatment worked when your body was resolving the problem on its own anyway. It can be coincidental that the pain resolved or improved after any medication or therapy. It happens more often than you might realize. Deciphering if the *brain* or the *body* needs assistance can be tricky but by addressing one you can typically help the other. After all, your "*br-ody*" comes in one package. For purposes of familiarity and organization, I will separate the professionals who can help you with pain as: *body* assistants and *brain* assistants.

Body Assistants

Again, medications or invasive treatments may mask the pain or blunt the signal that your body is relaying to your brain, but it is *not* always *fixing* the problem. Thus, your body mechanics and connective tissue are important issues to consider, and your pain is usually just reflecting asymmetries, imbalance or a non-neutral state for you. Your pain may self-resolve, or you may need some help. That is where a body assistant can come in handy. The trick is to figure out the problem or process that is contributing to your pain. The true problem may not be a single structure, and the brain's interpretation of the painful location may be misleading—perhaps your nervous system is the only one to blame.

Using fancy technology to create an image of the painful part can be helpful, but not always. Many people believe that taking pictures with an X-ray or an MRI is sufficient, but that does not necessarily give you all of the information of how your body moves. Imagine trying to assess the function of your brain with just a picture. Nowadays, there are functional MRIs (fMRIs) that give more active data to correlate with the patient's brain blood flow. This gives some indication of areas that are active during certain activities or situations. Even though this is not a complete explanation of exactly how the brain works, it is more data than a black and white static brain image found with traditional MRIs. Since the availability, affordability, and questionable adequacy limits the ability to assess musculoskeletal biomechanics via fMRIs, then a body mechanics expert can be helpful in correlating your body's condition with your symptoms.

Your body is truly a structure with many opposing forces. When does the moving structure of your body not matter in a world of gravity? It must be emphasized that "body mechanics" has an importance—yet, most physicians are not trained to understand this aspect of treatment. If a physician does not know how to detect a biomechanical problem, then how would a physician recognize the issue, least of all offer an appropriate solution? Consequently, it comes as less of a surprise that physicians may not be aware of the details or differences among various health professionals who perform or instruct patients on movement or manual therapies. And there are many who would argue that there is no good evidence that manual exams or therapies are reliable or effective; yet people can and have benefited. Therein lies the challenge of trying to find the appropriate *body assistant* for your pain.

First of all, what do I mean by a *body assistant*? Most of the professionals that help individuals with their body by *direct* treatment are called *bodyworkers*. I also like to refer to them as *body assistants* since they are *assisting* you with better movements and education, not just directly treating you. You could say that the previous chapter includes *body assistants* as well, but usually they can be easily accessed in a distant or group setting, not just individually. This chapter *primarily* relates to one-on-one treatments or assistance for pain within the medical or other health setting.

Most patients are familiar with the traditional physicians in America who can specialize in or treat pain. The first four are physicians that can become fellowship-trained as "pain medicine physicians":

- Anesthesiologist (M.D. or D.O.)
- Physiatrist [Physical Medicine and Rehabilitation Physician] (M.D. or D.O.)
- Neurologist (M.D. or D.O.)
- Psychiatrist (M.D. or D.O.)
- Podiatrist (D.P.M., only for foot/ankle pain), officially organized in the 1890s
- Osteopathic Manipulative Medicine Specialist (D.O.), since 1890s

Almost every specialty in medicine can deal with patients who have some sort of pain. Gynecologists can deal with female patients who have pelvic pain. Gastroenterologists can deal with patients who have abdominal pain. Rheumatologists can deal with patients who have rheumatoid arthritis. Hematologists can deal with patients diagnosed with sickle cell disease. Moreover, of course, primary care physicians can deal with any pain.

Some of the most common *non-physician* specialists who treat or help with pain:

- Physician Assistant (since 1960s), some with pain training
- Nurse Practitioner (since 1960s), some with pain training
- Physical Therapist, aka Physiotherapist (since 1910s)
- Occupational Therapist (since 1910s)
- Chiropractor (since 1890s)
- Osteopath (if not an osteopathic physician)
- Massage Therapist
- Personal Trainer
- Athletic Trainer
- Yoga Therapist

Below is an abbreviated version of some of the different body approaches or techniques, most of which are *not* performed by physicians. Despite minimal to moderate evidence currently available for their effectiveness for pain, many people find them useful with relatively little risk. They have the potential to affect the body in many ways including biomechanics, connective tissue, and/or the nervous system.

- Massage therapy
- Osteopathy/Osteopathic manipulative medicine[210,211]
- Strength training
- Stretching, static or dynamic
- Joint manipulation/mobilization
- Spinal manipulation/mobilization
- Chiropractic
- McKenzie Method
- Muscle energy techniques

- Myofascial release
- Acupuncture (slightly invasive with needles)
- Acupressure
- Active Release Therapy®
- Egoscue®
- Airrosti®
- Selective Functional Movement Assessment (SFMA)
- Neurostructural integration technique
- Bowen therapy
- Rolfing®
- Reiki
- Quantum Neurology®
- Electro-stimulation therapies
- Kraus 21-exercise method for back pain
- Traction
- Prolotherapy

Medical professionals can use many of these techniques and others not mentioned. **The more tools at a practitioner's disposal, then the more the approach can be uniquely tailored to each patient.** Regardless of technique, it is likely that treatment options and approaches will vary even within one specialty. For instance, if you put two physical therapists side-by-side, their approach will rarely be the same with the same patient. If you put two chiropractors side-by-side, their approaches can differ as well. In other words, not all medical professionals will approach the same patient the same way. This sounds oddly similar to how physicians approach the same problem with a slightly different twist. Differing approaches are not bad; in fact, it may be helpful. Also keep in mind, depending on how long your pain has been present, it could be more challenging to unravel the issues once you find the ideal caring and helpful provider.

Some of the techniques above, such as the Selective Functional Movement Assessment (SFMA), help look at the *overall* picture of the body's system in order to break down the *dysfunctional* movement patterns, which are not always related to the patient's complaint. Yet, the approach can lead to a more efficient and effective way to get to the *root cause* to better resolve the patient's pain. What I find most interesting about SFMA is that it addresses dysfunctions of *1)joint mobility, 2)tissue mobility and 3)stability/motor control*, which are reflective of the areas in which I find most physicians deficient: *1)biomechanics, 2)connective tissue, and 3)the nervous system*. In essence, the same issues with different wording.

However, the benefit to the SFMA methodical evaluation is that any interested practitioner can learn it to help evaluate the areas of *non-painful dysfunction* which may be contributing to pain elsewhere. After a full assessment, then the medical professional can use his or her own unique techniques or skills to address the perceived problem. The caveat is that *inexperienced* practitioners without skills for subtle observations may evaluate a patient with the SFMA when the patient is ill-suited for a standardized approach.

Regardless, your access to any of these treatment options are limited to what your insurance will cover, who is in your insurance network, what you can afford personally, or who is available in your home region. Sometimes these issues can be the most frustrating aspects of finding help for your pain, aside from figuring out what your problem is and who to see. However, you should still make the effort to seek resources online or in person. The Resources section at the back of this book provides some ideas for locating body assistants.

Why so much fragmentation of body assistants?

There is no manual that comes with the human body. I know I have mentioned this before, but it is essential that you keep this fact in mind. Humans have been trying to figure out the human body since the beginning of time. Different individuals or groups have claimed their methods help patients with pain. Whether the patient was going to improve despite the treatment or the treatment truly relieved the pain, the success stories put that particular profession in good stead with patients. Indeed, different approaches have evolved over time and lead to others branching off and claiming they have a different or more effective means of helping others with their pain or health issues.

For example, Andrew Taylor Still, an M.D. in the late 1800s, was fed up with the M.D.s *toxic* approaches to health such as bloodletting (removing blood as treatment). Thus, Dr. Still began studying how the musculoskeletal system was intimately related to pain and disease. Hence, osteopathy was born and the Doctor of Osteopathy degree began around the turn of the 20th century. Interestingly, not too long after Dr. Still shared his discoveries with others, D.D. Palmer became the "founder" of chiropractic. However, his son B.J. Palmer, was educated in the world of business and trained under his father to learn chiropractic, which eventually resulted in B.J. Palmer becoming the "developer" of chiropractic.[212] Despite denying training by the osteopathic medicine founder, Palmer wrote in 1899 per papers held at the Palmer College of Chiropractic:

> *Some years ago I took an expensive course in Electropathy, Cranial Diagnosis, Hydrotherapy, Facial Diagnosis. Later I took Osteopathy [which] gave me such a measure of confidence as to almost feel it unnecessary to seek other sciences for the mastery of curable disease. Having been assured that the underlying philosophy of chiropractic is the same as that of osteopathy... Chiropractic is osteopathy gone to seed.*[213,214]

It is not surprising that chiropractic has some similarities to osteopathy, but with different terms describing similar phenomena. No need to get in a turf war, but chiropractic has done a stronger job to infiltrate the mainstream with its business acumen. Osteopathy in the United States remains less well known, even though all osteopathic medical students spend hundreds of hours learning a variety of assessments and techniques to help those with pain or other ailments. Unfortunately, many osteopathic physicians choose medical careers or specialties that may not utilize those skills. However, osteopaths and some osteopathic physicians continue to hone and utilize their skills as the primary focus of their profession.

I envision that one day all physicians in medical school, whether M.D. or D.O., will have a better appreciation for the dynamic, not static, aspects of the human body and be able to appreciate, diagnose, educate, and/or treat the asymmetries or dysfunctions of the body that may lead to or cause pain.

Society can benefit from learning "the best of the best" regardless of which profession. Each profession is dabbling with trying to understand and help humans, especially those who suffer from pain. In addition, until we have the "pain thing" perfected, physicians, non-physicians, and patients could learn a lot from one another.

How do you navigate through the body assistants?

The approach is rational and not any different from previous discussions on opioids and invasive procedures—maximize the benefits while reducing the risks.

- If you are in a tender, "jumpy," or "wound-up" state of pain, then there can be an increased potential of worsening pain with *aggressive* therapies.
    - Calming the nervous system with meditation, acupuncture, or gentle techniques can be attempted prior to progressing.
    - On rare occasion, pain medications or procedures may be used temporarily to calm an exquisitely sensitive nervous system to allow for more effective manual or movement therapy by a body assistant.
- If the body assistant is able to provoke mechanical pain in a reproducible way, then this could suggest musculoskeletal or biomechanical sources of pain.
    - Finding an expert who can treat reversible issues is worth investigating.
    - Pain that can be provoked may help the body assistant guide you on smarter movements that do not set your body up for injury.
    - At the very least, discovering how to maintain optimal stability versus flexibility may help prevent dysfunction or pain.
- Non-painful, gentle approaches should be attempted first, if appropriate.
    - Patient-directed, patient-assisted, or provider-directed manual therapies are examples of maneuvers that use lower velocities to effect change in your body.
    - Gentle and small changes may require more treatments to ensure adequate and lasting effects.

- Popping or quick thrust maneuvers, such as on the spine, tend to incorporate a velocity that could potentially injure you or exacerbate your pain, but this is rare.
    - Osteoporosis can increase the risk of fracture with these maneuvers.
    - Use as a last resort or for obvious recent acute changes, such as a shoulder dislocation.
    - The rare risk of vertebral artery dissection can occur with poorly executed "neck popping."
- You should also **receive education** in certain activities or exercises that will help you guide or maintain symmetry or homeostasis for long-term benefit.
    - Without education, you can become dependent or passive in the process if it is a chronic or recurring issue. Understanding what provokes pain can help you avoid pain without limiting function.
    - In light of escalating health care costs, this world is only getting more populated, with more demands on the health care system, and you would be better served by learning how to take care of yourself with some professional guidance.
- The length or number of treatments depends on how long your pain has been around and/or your response to treatments.
    - If your mind and body have been accustomed to chronic pain signals, then it may take some time to calm down the nervous system and unravel the issues.
    - There typically needs to be more consistency in efforts secondary to the interconnectedness of the body, tissue adaptability, and brain adaptability.
    - If your body took a while to get to a place of pain, then it may take longer than you want to reverse it.
    - It can take time for a body assistant to understand your body and its responses to treatment, as not all bodies are made exactly the same. Hips, for example, can vary structurally.

- Consider a different approach or practitioner if multiple similar efforts or treatments are not giving at least some reasonable improvement in your function or pain.
    - Even if there is still some pain or soreness but you notice some element of improved range of motion or a slight ease in movement after your activity or treatment, then that is usually a good sign.
    - Sometimes, too much treatment can be harmful or unnecessary; yet, too little or inappropriate treatment can be unhelpful as well.
    - Suggestion by a body assistant for a standard number or excessive treatments (e.g., 30 sessions) *without* mention of reassessing the body's unique response to treatment should raise concern. Patients can be vulnerable to over-selling by alternative or complementary medicine businesses as well.
    - Maintain a dialogue and always re-assess if moving in a positive direction.

Better movement typically helps the pain signal dampen. Days to weeks of continued effort can lead to a positive change in your pain. Remember, the longer the pain has been around, the more important it is to do preventive maintenance. **Self-care must never be discarded. It is always important regardless if you have pain or not. Self-care can also prevent pain; just as eating healthy and exercising can prevent diabetes. You have already proven that you are susceptible or vulnerable to acquire the pain—so, keep it at bay! Make the effort. A better quality of life is worth it.**

Speak with your physician or search your community's resources for *body assistants* to help you get to a better place of balance in your body to enable the *possibility* of a pain-free life or at least less pain. This can be an extremely challenging part of the pain journey—finding the ideal body assistant. Find someone who will persistently seek answers or solutions, or at the very least, refer you to someone else who will not give up on you! Even if a specific *cause* of your pain cannot be pinpointed, there are healthy ways to approach pain that may help even if the "why" or "how" of those approaches are unclear.

Brain Assistants

> *All pain has a psychological component and psychological factors are important at all stages of pain (whether the problem is acute, recurrent or chronic) and have a major role in the prevention of unnecessary pain-associated dysfunction in a wide range of settings from primary prevention to terminal care.*
>
> —**International Association for the Study of Pain**, 1997

Remember, you cannot experience pain without your physically present *brain*. Your awareness and interpretation of your circumstances is one of the ways in which your *mind* can exert some influence on that brain.

Although there are many ways you can help your brain with the food you eat, the exercise you do, the meditation you do, or the environment to which you subject yourself, it can be helpful to have a coach to support you in acquiring additional perspective and skills to optimize your mind's management of the pain. In the United States, various health professionals can assist you with any psychological issues that may be hindering your optimal management of pain:

- Psychologists
- Social workers
- Psychiatric nurses
- Psychiatrists
- Physician assistants
- Nurse practitioners
- Yoga therapists

Psychiatrists, physician assistants, and some nurse practitioners are the only ones legally licensed to prescribe medications; however, starting with the lowest risk and most empowering option of *mental skills* is a practical place to start with all of the brain assistants. Just like other specialties, there will always be certain professionals who are quick to write prescriptions, despite a lack of serious or unstable psychiatric issues. Look for someone who has training in pain, if possible. There are a variety of techniques that can be utilized not only for patients in pain but those with underlying anxiety and depression, whether it started before or because of the pain.

One of the most heavily supported methods in the world of pain is **cognitive behavioral therapy**. It is an effective method for helping patients with pain, anxiety, depression, post-traumatic stress disorder, and obsessive-compulsive disorder. By examining thoughts, feelings, and behaviors, the brain assistant can help the patient recognize the connection of negative thoughts to negative feelings, which can lead to self-sabotaging behaviors. Many times the patient will be challenged to examine and demonstrate that their thoughts, such as "I am worthless" or "I am going to hurt my back more," are not truths but beliefs that are not real.

These negative beliefs can lead to depression or *learned helplessness*. In the 1960s, a psychologist Dr. Martin Seligman and his colleagues performed a study to assess fear and learning in dogs. The dog was allowed to escape an area after hearing a tone and receiving a non-damaging shock. Yet, after placing that same dog in an enclosure with two areas divided by a low fence, the dog did not bother to evade the shock whether or not the tone occurred. In fact, the dog would just lie down. Yet, if a dog that was not trained to associate the tone with shock was put into the fenced off compartments, then that dog would immediately jump over the fence to escape the shock. Despite learning that a tone accompanied a shock, the *conditioned* dog felt as if it was futile to avoid the shock and accepted the pain. This learned helplessness seems very similar to humans who are depressed in environments where circumstances seem unchangeable and the drive to make an effort seems extinguished.[215] Learned helplessness seems to emerge with chronic pain patients when efforts to eliminate pain are unsuccessful.

Whether there are emotional or physical challenges in life, we all react to them in different and unique ways. It is common for helplessness, depression, or hopelessness to consume any of us if vulnerable enough and if the body and mind are not supported appropriately. Some of us are more susceptible to pessimistic vantage points than others. As an example, one person can be "dumped" in an emotional relationship and be sad only briefly while another can be devastated and unable to see anything positive in life for an extended period of time. Emotional pain combined with a negative perspective can create tremendous suffering. Likewise, physical pain can strain the brain in a variety of ways.

If there is any question as to how profoundly pain and the surrounding environment can affect an individual, then take a moment to read this pain sufferer's eloquent statement found in the frequently referenced Institute of Medicine's *Relieving Pain in America* report:

> *The impersonal hostility of the payment system, the intellectual poverty of the research, and the cognitive poverty of my providers, combined to turn me from a spirited and capable professional with a good income and a bright future, into a needy dependent of the state with no profession, no future, and a life that is ever more bleak and limited by pain, weakness, disenchantment, and despair.*

Sadly, many people find their life turned upside down because of unrelenting pain. It leads some patients to suicide. If you have any thoughts of hurting yourself or others, please get help. Regardless of where your mind is in all of this pain, it is even more reason to utilize different sources of guidance. There is help within and outside the traditional medical field for optimizing your own *body*, *mind*, and *spirit* to minimize the suffering that can come with pain. By working on at least one of those areas, it can help give you the strength to work on the other areas and lift you out of despair. But first **you need someone to truly listen to you**.

It is common to seek out a "cure" for your pain, but many areas of you are affected. Merely looking for the bodily cause of your pain while ignoring or minimizing the importance of your mind or brain can ironically make your pain worse. Despite your legitimate search for the *cause* of your pain, do yourself a favor and keep that brain from progressing into a more wound-up state than necessary. Do all that you can do to keep your nervous system calmer with your personal mindfulness practices or the assistance from a brain assistant. Should you find a bodily cause, it will make it easier and faster for those who *can* help you with your pain, if your nervous system has been kept in check. The resources at the end of this book may give you some places to look or start your path to a more skillful mind and healthier brain with less pain.

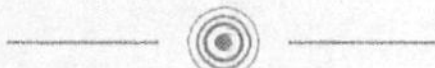

Aiming for no pain sounds ideal, but the reality is life consists of some level of physical or emotional pain from time to time. Learning how to put pain into perspective or manage it are the keys to success. Ultimately, the goal is to find body and brain assistants who acknowledge and practice with an understanding that multiple areas of your life and different aspects of your body can be affected by or contribute to pain. Remember, the body and brain are really part of *one* system, the "*br-ody*," which is affected by internal *and* external factors.

CHAPTER 22

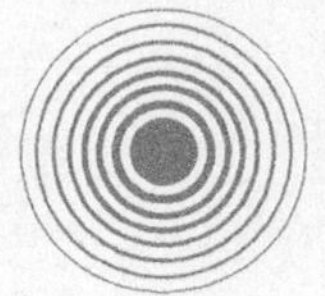

Get Off the Pain Train!

I advocate for a totally new view of the role of the patient: patient as engaged partner, not passive recipient.

—**Dave deBronkart**, *e-Patient Dave*

If you are in pain, then your physician may give you a diagnosis—whether accurate or not. There are common medications and procedures that will be offered to you by a traditional pain physician based on that diagnosis. Yes, pain physicians can help some people improve or resolve their pain. Yet, if you choose indiscriminately without trying to understand what and why certain things are being done, then you are at risk for getting on the "pain train." In this profit-driven medical system, be careful what you ask for. You will likely get what you want and more, whether you need it or not.

If you do not realize that an injection is meant to *diagnose* which nerve is sending the information toward your brain, then you may think that the injection is a cure for your inactivity or some other body mechanics problem. That "diagnostic" injection may only give a few hours of relief. You could go down a path of multiple injections until a decision is made to burn the nerves so that you can get longer relief. Because of burning the nerve, you may have months of relief but the nearby muscles served by those burned nerves will weaken. If no personal effort is made to improve your own body, then the pain train continues. If you remain a passive participant and do not attempt to work on self-care or get some other assessments of your overall body mechanics and connective tissue, then you are on a perpetual pain train.

My best recommendation is to look at managing your pain with *pain bridges*, not pain trains. Pain physicians will have medications, injections, and other modalities to offer you. They usually have a small window of time to spend with you. Medications are the quickest to offer, but they should be used to help facilitate movement and therapies, hence pain bridges. If they do not help you do that, then you should discuss with your physician whether it is worthwhile to continue. Staying on that train may not make much *sense*—only *cents* out of your pocket. More invasive interventions should be looked at the same way. If they are not helping you achieve a more functional life, then re-evaluate with your physician. Most pain physicians will encourage other manual or movement therapies if helpful, but there are varying perspectives and opinions out there with respect to their effectiveness. The more you complain and demand *unnecessary* interventions, the more the business of medicine profits *unnecessarily*.

If pain were more straightforward, then there would not be such variability in opinions. What pain physicians offer you has the potential to make you passive, if you choose to be. If you do not take action to help yourself, then you will be more dependent on that medical provider. If you want to live the rest of your life with fewer visits to a physician, especially a pain physician, then you must become more involved with your own care. **If you look at medical interventions as "bridges" to help facilitate the things you should be doing for yourself, then you will be more successful than not.** Taking more pain medication without improving your activity or function is not enabling your body to be better from the inside out. There must be a personal effort to cause truly sustainable, healthy change.

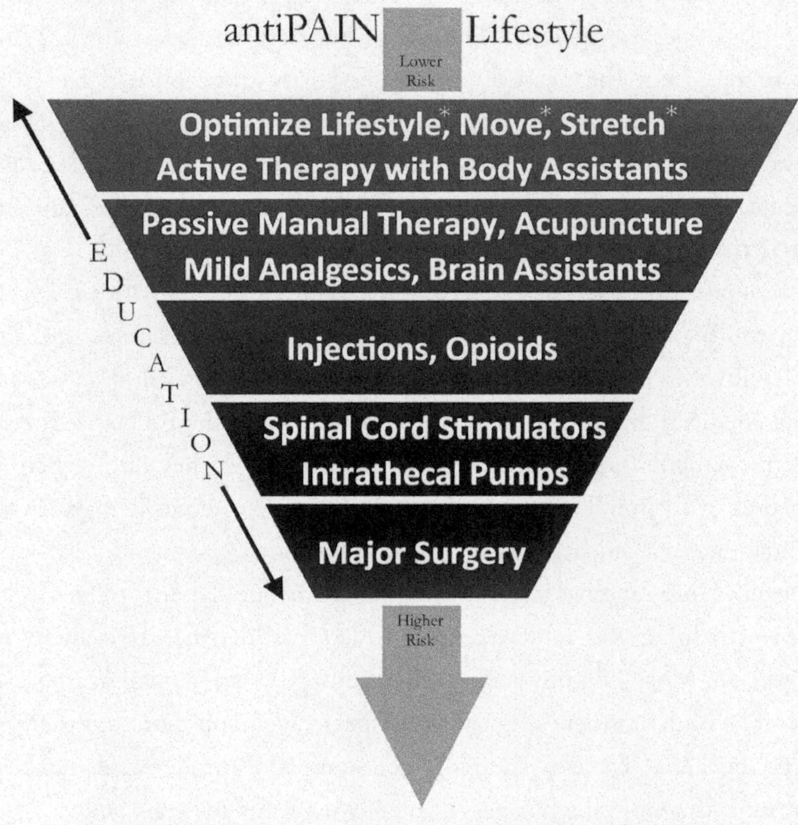

Figure 19: **The antiPAIN Lifestyle**. After ruling out red flags, the priority is to optimize one's self with healthy habits. The progression of assistance should always start with less risky and less invasive interventions. Based on the unique situation, some of the more invasive interventions may actually be less risky for an individual (e.g., spinal cord stimulator versus opioids), but this is a general idea for progression. Reassessment and re-evaluation for emerging red flags is implied. **Education should be pursued at all stages of the pain journey.**

Today, it is quite common to treat *symptoms* and not the *cause* in medicine. Ideally, treating symptoms should be for acute situations or brief periods to allow for healing or for enabling easier therapy or better function. **In other words, use addictive medications or invasive procedures as a last resort or as a bridge to accomplishing self-care.** (see Figure 19) **Otherwise, you are unwittingly becoming dependent on others to treat the symptoms and relinquishing some or all of the power that you have to modify or control your own pain experience.** There is still risk with injections and procedures despite advanced technology. If you are receiving heavy sedation for procedures, then you are adding another layer of risk. Most people do fine with heavy sedation for these procedures, but it can be tricky with some patients who have significant medical issues, including heart disease, lung disease, significant obesity, sleep apnea, etc.

Most patients pursue medications, injections, and surgeries, because they just want the pain to go away. I cannot blame them. You may feel that you have been given a legitimate diagnosis or reason for having the intervention. When patients receive injections, why do they get better briefly or indefinitely?

- Was it perfectly timed to when the patient was going to get better anyway?
- Was there a placebo effect so the brain believed it would get better?
- Was the intervention helping for reasons other than what was intended?
- Did it break the pain cycle to allow the body a chance to move better?
- Did it just calm the nervous system?

When a patient elects to have back surgery when there is no concerning radiculopathy or other serious pathology, is it possible the patient could have improved without surgery?

- Did the surgery help mainly because the patient finally got serious about physical therapy after surgery and knew they needed to work through the postoperative pain, which in this case was considered *normal and expected*?

- Did the one or more hours of retractors stretching the muscles and other connective tissue do the trick more than the lumbar fusion surgery?
- Was the lumbar fusion creating stability that could have been accomplished with more appropriate biomechanical training?

These are all good questions with no easy answers.

Is it acceptable to continue to want an answer to your pain? Yes. This may be in direct conflict with many colleagues who believe the patient should accept the pain and learn how to deal with it. Let me clarify. I believe it is acceptable for a patient to want to understand his or her condition better, but *not at the expense of ignoring self-care or learning the skills to down-regulate one's own nervous system.*

Catastrophizing or overly fixating on finding out the cause of your pain can intensify the areas in the brain perceiving pain. Magnifying your pain in your brain is not helpful. At the same time, covering pain with drugs or burning nerves could inadvertently complicate or possibly increase the pain signals if there is something correctable, whether we understand it now or it is something yet to be discovered.

Let's think of a simplistic example. If a demented, elderly man had a splinter in his toe but does not remember an episode of anything contacting his foot nor is it visible to the naked eye, then it is very possible that further investigation may not be pursued. The new and associated anxiety or pain symptoms in the demented patient may be treated with medications. Yet, if the splinter was removed, then those symptoms would not have existed, making it unnecessary to treat the pain or the anxiety.

If better approaches are used to address the *cause*, then the pain could be reversed or decreased. It took six different physicians to help me understand why I had low back pain. It may not have been an exact or precise answer but something was not in balance and there were certain manual modalities that helped *bridge* me from extreme pain and decreased function to no pain and full function. Through this process, I learned to pay attention to what was aggravating my low back and pelvis. I was no longer a victim. Putting the power of managing pain in the patient's hands creates a less dependent patient, *if the patient is motivated.* Most patients inherently know that their care should be personalized, but they may not think of it in those words. Many times it comes out in the form of:

- "The doctor thinks it is all in my head,"
- "They never touched me or examined me," or
- "But I don't want to take pain medication."

If you are still in pain or having trouble coping with the pain, then never underestimate the importance of getting professional help. Finding the right patient advocate can assist or *bridge* you with becoming your own master at self-regulating your brain and body to decrease your pain. You need skills that can help you help yourself—ultimately, *to get off the pain train*. Challenge yourself to modify your brain's perception of pain while you are seeking a possible answer and improving your self-care. Physicians, body and brain assistants, *and you* can help you conquer your pain and minimize the suffering. Now that you understand the complexity of this *Paindemic*, **what you DO know can HELP you!**

CHAPTER 23

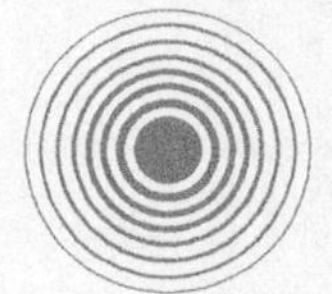

How Can WE Control This Paindemic?

To raise new questions, new possibilities, to regard old problems from a new angle, requires creative imagination and marks real advance in science.
—Albert Einstein

Throughout this book, I made a case for why this *Paindemic* exists. We know that if we address a single patient's pain using opioids, then we mask the symptoms. Intuitively, we know society is approaching this nation's *Paindemic* in a similar manner. To treat the growing epidemic of overdose deaths by expanding access to opioid reversal agents and punishing physicians for prescribing opioids are putting bandages on the underlying problems. Well-intentioned physicians need more knowledge and options to help their patients in pain and society needs a paradigm shift. As a nation, we need to get on the same page and do more than treat symptoms!

None of us were handed the true manual of the human body by the manufacturer, whoever you believe that to be. Yes, medicine has come a long way such as treating infections or saving trauma victims, but this developed country has not conquered the infectious mentality that we must always have an *immediate* answer and never be uncomfortable! Understanding and educating about the pain challenge is seriously lacking in this country.

Not looking for a cause of pain is a form of negligence, *but only if the provider is aware of the issues likely contributing to pain.* Unfortunately, traditional medical schools do not have a reliable curriculum to determine the cause of prevalent pain, such as low back pain. Osteopathic medical schools do give some helpful training in osteopathic manipulative medicine, but many of those graduates do not use those skills in their practice. We need to update curriculums in all medical schools (M.D. and D.O.) regarding the less understood realms of our bodies, including biomechanics, connective tissue, and the nervous system.

In addition to osteopathic medicine, multiple other health care professionals have impressive understanding and skills for addressing the body's biomechanics, connective tissue, and nervous system. In fact, their intuition and abilities are hard to understand by casual observers and difficult to validate in large studies. In the end, everything in the "body system" works synergistically. Each part cannot survive in isolation. Ignoring or discounting the importance of a part of that body system assumes that it is unnecessary or unimportant. By doing this, we can be overlooking a potentially important contribution to a patient's pain. Yes, we need to see the forest for the trees.

Currently, there is a strong push to use interdisciplinary approaches to pain management, which is most appropriate for when we have difficulty figuring out *why* there is pain or when it appears unfixable. With inadequate education for most physicians regarding biomechanics, connective tissue, and the neurologic basis of pain, incorporating a collaborative approach to the patient's pain is likely to offer greater benefits and reinforces how many of us have different tools and perspectives. No need for turf wars among specialties; too many patients need help and the best care possible. It is better to have more minds involved, but it should always begin with lower risk options once the red flags are ruled out.

There is also a growing trend in the medical field to focus on weaning off opioids and learning to "cope" with the pain but without any guidance or efforts to incorporate the *body*. Just as the physical body is not the only contributor to pain, the brain is not the sole contributor to the experience of pain. The brain and body interact with one another intimately. Thus, multiple non-invasive *body* approaches also should be attempted early, not after trying out multiple surgeries in hopes of giving relief. Once unnecessary surgeries happen, the body has been altered in a way that may be difficult to treat and could lead to a cascade of other compensations that could contribute to more pain. So much more money and time is spent putting patients through these procedures and surgeries, but the patient continues to hold on to the hope that the next surgery will fix the problem. If you are on the fifth back surgery with no obvious red flag and nothing has helped, then the medical field needs to encourage you to stop banging your head against the wall and realize that there must be less taxing approaches. Chronic pain is not typically *life-threatening*! It is *life altering* and can consume you, but you are better off pursuing safer alternatives first.

Knowing that pain is usually a sign something is wrong, covering up the pain with medications or unnecessary procedures can just delay addressing the primary issue. The pain becomes more entrenched and complicated as the body tries to compensate in multiple ways. It makes it harder to discern the original contributor or cause of pain. The pain cycle is perpetuated in this way. A physician may need to engage various disciplines sooner than later to avoid the initiation of opioids or other invasive procedures. Those riskier options should be used as *bridges* to improve function not as a *train* to keep the patient on, if at all possible. It is easier for physicians to prescribe opioids, but it is incredibly difficult to stop the medications after the patient starts taking them. In addition, it is sometimes difficult for the patient to acknowledge that the non-drug, non-invasive approach is actually helping if the picture is blurred or complicated by the use of opioids.

By treating the symptoms, you cover up the very issue that is telling you that the cause is not being addressed. But, herein lies the problem. The lack of training and appreciation for biomechanics, connective tissue, and nervous system in medical training exists; thus, physicians have fewer tools in the toolbox.

Many physicians, especially pain medicine physicians, will typically reinforce not trying to find the cause, as the patient needs to learn how to cope with the pain they already have with medications, injections and other more invasive, risky therapies in which those physicians are highly trained.

The stumbling block is trying to convince misguided patients that the original "diagnosis" or treatment may be incorrect or inappropriate. This is especially difficult if the first opinion comes from a provider who the patient trusts wholeheartedly. It can also come from a provider who has a strong financial incentive to do an intervention to the patient or is not open-minded enough for less invasive options to address the possible cause. As medical professionals, they should do no harm. One must question the excessive injections and drugs if the physician or patient did not put in a strong and consistent effort toward the noninvasive approaches. Patients need better education.

Even more challenging is when the patient already has had physical therapy or chiropractic work done with unsatisfactory results. *Not* all body assistants are the same. There is an art involved. Sometimes it takes more detective work or different approaches within the realm of conservative care. Patients must understand this reality.

Humans are not cars. They are living, adaptable, and amazing beings that deserve to be treated as such and not as an object on the medical assembly line. I've heard time and again from providers that it is all about the safety of the patient and helping their pain, but everyone is not stepping back to look at the big picture. Patients accept more risk than necessary. **Rational approaches must be driven into clinical practice to avoid unintentionally misguiding patients down a path of unnecessary drugs, injections, and surgery.**

We all know that today's society tends to seek the quick fix. Physicians are making the "symptom" approach too convenient, despite their compassion for helping those in pain. Drugs are easier to dish out than emphasizing the need to address the small habits that may be leading the patient into more pain. Do physicians really want to keep treating symptoms forever and making patients passive in their life? It is costly for the patient and for society. If money is the primary driver, then yes, passive patients create a form of consistent income for medical professionals or facilities.

Ultimately, this country needs *collaboration*. We all play roles. As the saying goes, it takes a village. As patients, do the little things to live the antiPAIN Lifestyle. As caregivers, encourage, give hope, and avoid enabling the patient. As medical professionals, listen, educate and rule out the true emergencies or urgencies and help facilitate the least risk when interventions are necessary. As researchers, continue to pursue an understanding of connective tissue, biomechanics, the nervous system, and beyond so that the medical world can better appreciate the inherent intelligence of the body's system. As educators, continue to adapt the medical school curriculum to reflect evolving understandings of the human body. As for anyone who is greedy at the expense of a patient's health, there is no room for it in this health care system. All of this may be a tall order, but in the future, we may be able to provide better and more affordable strategies to improve the function and quality of our lives with less or *no* pain!

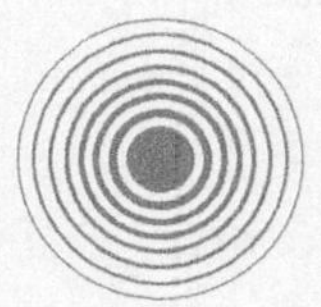

Speak Up! There is HOPE!

There is a saying in Tibetan. "Tragedy should be utilized as a source of strength." No matter what sort of difficulties, how painful experience is, if we lose our hope, that's our real disaster.

—Dalai Lama XIV

I feel that one of the biggest injustices to patients is eliminating any hope they have for pain relief, without medications or invasive interventions. I am so glad I did not give up on seeking the cause of my pain or finding noninvasive ways to manage it. Most of my colleagues do not understand how I take care of my back or what I do to immediately resolve an acute bout of low back pain. In all fairness, physicians only know what they have been taught, but there is no doubt that most of them genuinely want their patients to feel better. However, more data and stories are needed to prove the antiPAIN Lifestyle works.

My hope is that readers of this book do not become *diagnocentric* because this society focuses on immediate gratification and self-entitlement. Regardless of the diagnoses or labels the health care system uses, everyone has the power to be their "best" self. Health care professionals should be facilitators of a collaborative process based on the patient's values and what is best for that patient's health. Patients may not like what physicians say, but sometimes the best advocates let them know what they need to hear. Some patients will need more help than others will, but in the end, everyone has only one body to live in. Making it the best it can be will provide for a lifetime of gratitude.

I love to hear transformations of friends, family, and patients that move from a life of pain to one of less or no pain. I encourage you to **share your story at www.PainOutLoud.com** so that others can believe there are healthy and effective ways of approaching pain—and more importantly, give others hope. If you believe your physician is open to reading this book, then recommend it or give it to your physician so that they can help you and others who may be dealing with pain by adopting an additional perspective. We must overcome this *Paindemic* and you can help by helping yourself and others.

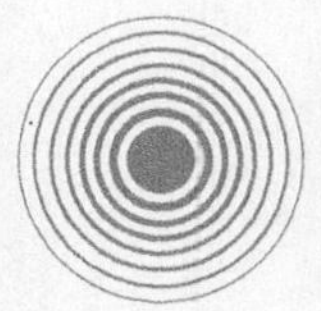

Afterword

Many patients are not told that or do not readily comprehend, that the road to finding the right combination of treatments for them, may be a long one with many different approaches to treatment until the right match is found.
— **Institute of Medicine**, *Relieving Pain in America*

The existence of this *Paindemic* reveals many questions that remain to be answered. Other fields outside of the pain world have recognized the value and the importance of an interdisciplinary approach to some of the most challenging of health issues. Thus, pain medicine has vast room for improvement among the current medical specialties. The promise of the pain world's future depends on patients, educators, researchers, and health care professionals regardless of *classification* or *title*. **There is a dire need for collaboration and effective and expeditious communication among one another regarding assessment and diagnosis, not just treatment of chronic**

pain. Regulatory and governmental agencies should uphold moral and ethical obligations and not hinder these genuine efforts. In doing the *right* thing, we can more effectively increase the function and quality of life for many people living in pain. *Patients* are an essential part to the discovery and evolution of society's knowledge of pain. Most people at some time or another will experience pain—it knows no boundaries. Thus, this national reality is a global obligation to diminish the burden and suffering of this *Paindemic*.

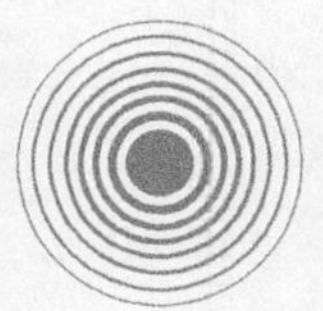

About the Author

Melissa Cady, D.O. is an osteopathic physician schooled extensively in the traditional medical field. She completed a variety of training after medical school: one year of general surgery, one year of internal medicine, three years of anesthesiology training, and one year of pain medicine fellowship training. Because of her training and exams, she is currently board certified in anesthesiology and pain medicine by the American Board of Anesthesiology. She currently practices in Austin, Texas.

Dr. Cady did her undergraduate work at the University of Texas at Austin receiving a Bachelor of Science in Microbiology degree. In her senior year, she worked at physical therapy clinics and doctors' offices gaining knowledge from the clinical and business sides of medicine.

Dr. Cady also ran a part-time personal training business before and during medical school. Her continued passion for fitness led her to winning the Fit Company's honor of "Fittest Doctor 2013" for Austin, Texas and "Fittest Doctor 2012" for San Antonio, Texas after rigorous competition. She enjoys being a *practical* role model and inspiring others to challenge their fitness and health.

Dr. Cady is a member of the American Osteopathic Association, Texas Osteopathic Medical Association, American Society of Anesthesiologists, Texas Society of Anesthesiologists, and Texas Pain Society. In addition, Dr. Cady has spent many hours mentoring students, writing articles, and giving presentations for the community regarding various medical and health issues.

Known as the "Challenge Doctor," Dr. Cady is driven to champion the cause of living the antiPAIN Lifestyle and minimizing the current *Paindemic* so rampant today. Her views are born from medical training and personal experience, as she has personally managed her own journey with pain in a safer and healthier manner than today's medical system would likely facilitate.

More information about Dr. Cady and requests for speaking engagements can be found on her personal website, **www.ChallengeDoctor.com.**

To share *your* story of how *you* found healthy ways to improve or overcome *your* own pain challenge, go to **www.PainOutLoud.com.**

Acknowledgments

This book journey has been filled with overwhelming excitement, enlightenment, edification, and encouragement. In reality, it began with a disenchantment of how the pain world currently exists and how I fit within it. I never really set out with the intent to write a book, but I knew too many people were suffering with pain in an irrational medical system. So, I began believing in my vision and shared my message with others. That belief began to be magnified by the support of so many wonderful people. They each played important roles.

If it was not for a random and insightful conversation with a gym-goer, Allen Kenroy, then I may not have started down the path of acknowledging my passion and writing *Paindemic*®. *Thank you for opening my eyes to the possibilities, Allen.*

Before and after embarking on book writing, I have been blessed by the tutelage and support of great teachers—some are physicians but many include non-physicians, including patients. Specifically for this book, I am in appreciation of Amanda Tuttle Thielen, Anagha Agte, Bennett Ezekiel, Betty and Richard Hinds, Brendon Burchard, Bryan Cady, Connie Speece Stanchek, Conrad Speece, Crystal Cameron, Debra Hathaway, Jamie Guyden, Jana Sanders, Janet Martin, Joy Whipple, Justin Fox, Kerri Brooker, Kery Feferman, Max Eckmann, Michelle Craven, Mike Chapoton, Neil Pearson, Rebecca Osborne, Rod Corbin,

Somayaji Ramamurthy, Sonya Gloier, Stuart McGill, Tracey Haas, and many of the unnamed people who have crossed my path to help make this book possible. Some of them didn't even know that they taught me or helped me in some way. *Thank you all.*

And a special appreciation is in order for Donna Grumbles, a friend who has taken on her own journey of suffering this past year. She has been a brave fighter despite multiple unexpected setbacks. Donna's relentless pursuit to optimize her own health, despite the challenges ahead, is what makes her a hero to all of us. *You are loved, Donna.*

And to my editor, Lisbeth "Lis" Tanz, who helped take this book to another level. Lis was able to tame my billowing enthusiasm and words from distracting the reader. Her advice and guidance were essential for embarking on my first book. *Thank you, Lis.*

And to Morgan James Publishing, of course, who embraced my book from the beginning to enable another outlet for my message. *Thank you for this wonderful opportunity.*

And thank you to Marsha Yearian, who is a woman of many talents, from Internet marketer to website designer to "Super Mom." She has been a compassionate supporter, guide, and friend to me since my mission's infancy. Marsha has genuinely believed in my vocation to inform the public of ways to challenge their lives for the better and decrease their pain. *I appreciate you more than you know, Marsha.*

And a special thank you to Dr. Roberto Ruiz and his wife Cindy who supported me unconditionally during my medical training. *Your generosity has never been forgotten.*

And a very special thank you to my parents, Armi and Bruce Cady, for bringing me into this amazing world and for their unconditional love, support, and contributions to this book. *I am proud of every effort you both make to challenge your health in a positive way. My love for both of you, Mom and Dad, is beyond measure.*

Last but not least, I am truly blessed by the *Love of My Life*, Corey Jackson. I could not ask for a more supportive, emotionally available, loving, understanding, and encouraging partner in my life. *I have learned more about myself because of you,*

Corey. And when I needed time for the book, you were willing to make the sacrifice with me. I am forever grateful for your steadfast commitment to our relationship in the wake of my fervent mission to minimize this Paindemic.

Notes

Chapter 1- *Paindemic*®: There is Pain Everywhere!

1 IOM (Institute of Medicine), *Relieving Pain in America: A Blueprint for Transforming Prevention, Care, Education, and Research* (Washington, DC: The National Academies Press, 2011).

2 Theo Vos et al, "Years Lived with Disability (YLDs) for 1160 Sequelae of 289 Diseases and Injuries 1990–2010: a Systematic Analysis for the Global Burden of Disease Study 2010," *Lancet* 380, no. 9859 (2012): 2163-96. doi:10.1016/S0140-6736(12)61729-2.

3 "Chronic Pain Rates Shoot Up Until Americans Reach Late 50s," last modified April 27, 2012, http://www.gallup.com/poll/154169/Chronic-Pain-Rates-Shoot-Until-Americans-Reach-Late-50s.aspx?utm_source=chronic%20pain%20rates&utm_medium=search&utm_campaign=tiles.

4 International Association for the Study of Pain, accessed March 8, 2015, http://www.iasp-pain.org/Taxonomy?navItemNumber=576.

5 Norman Doidge, *The Brain That Changes Itself: Stories of Personal Triumph from the Frontiers of Brain Science* (London: Penguin, 2007).

6 Alban Latremoliere and Clifford J Woolf, "Central Sensitization: A Generator of Pain Hypersensitivity by Central Neural Plasticity," *J Pain* 10 no.9 (2009): 895-926. doi:10.1016/j.jpain.2009.06.012.

7 Marion Lee et al, "A Comprehensive Review of Opioid-Induced Hyperalgesia," *Pain Physician* 14 (2011): 145-61.

8 Lars Arendt-Nielsen et al, "Viscero-Somatic Reflexes in Referred Pain Areas Evoked by Capsaicin Stimulation of the Human Gut," *European J Pain* 12, no.5 (2008): 544-51. doi:10.1016/j.ejpain.2007.08.010.

Chapter 2- Humans Don't Come with a Manual at Birth

9 David L. Katz, "God's Radio is Broken," last modified Jan 13, 2014, http://www.linkedin.com/today/post/article/201401131620-23027997-god-s-radio-is-broken?trk=eml-ced-b-art-M-0&ut=0JGaJs6zxtrC41.

10 Steven King, "Understanding Complex Regional Pain Syndrome," last modified May 23, 2013, http://www.consultantlive.com/pain-management/understanding-complex-regional-pain-syndrome.

11 Caldwell B. Esselstyn Jr., "Resolving the Coronary Artery Disease Epidemic Through Plant-Based Nutrition," *Preventive Cardiology* 4, no.4 (2001): 171-77.

12 Caldwell B. Esselstyn Jr. et al, "A Way to Reverse CAD?" *J Family Practice* 63, no.7 (2014): 356-364b.

Chapter 3- The Invisible Burden: Out of Sight Or *Out of Your Mind*?

13 International Association for the Study of Pain, accessed March 8, 2015, http://www.iasp-pain.org/Taxonomy?navItemNumber=576.

14 Joy Whipple, "Chronic Post-op Pain: A Clinician/Patient's Perspective," *Anesthesiology News* 39.5 (2013): 6.

Chapter 4- Your Body's Ability to Adapt & Heal

15 Thomas E. Strax et al, "Physical Modalities, Therapeutic Exercise, Extended Bedrest, and Aging Effects," in *Physical Medicine and Rehabilitation Board Review*, 2nd ed., ed. Thomas E. Strax et al. (New York: Demos Medical Publishing, 2009), 633.

16 Strax et al, "Physical Modalities," 634.

17 Dava Newman, "Humans in Space," Lecture given on Dec 8, 2009, accessed online on March 7, 2015. http://techtv.mit.edu/videos/16588-humans-in-space.

18 "Known Effects of Long-Term Space Flights on the Human Body," accessed online on March 7, 2015. http://www.racetomars.ca/mars/article_effects.jsp.

19 Robert Gailey et al, "Review of Secondary Physical Conditions Associated with Lower-Limb Amputation and Long-Term Prosthesis Use," *J Rehabilitation Research and Development* 45, no.1 (2008): 15-30.

20 Jai Kulkarni et al, "Chronic low back pain in traumatic lower limb amputees," *Clinical Rehabilitation* 19, no. 1 (2005): 81–86.

21 Thomas Buchheit, Thomas Van de Ven, and Andrew Shaw, "Epigenetics and the Transition from Acute to Chronic Pain," *Pain Medicine* 13, no.11 (2012): 1474-90. doi:10.1111/j.1526-4637.2012.01488.x.

Chapter 5- The Dilemma of Pain Avoidance

22 Tamar Pincus et al, "The Fear Avoidance Model Disentangled: Improving the Clinical Utility of the Fear Avoidance Model," *Clinical J Pain* 26, no.9 (2010): 739-46.

23 Neil Pearson, personal communication with author, March 20, 2015.

24 James Rainville et al, "Fear-Avoidance Beliefs and Pain Avoidance in Low Back Pain—Translating Research into Clinical Practice," *Spine Journal* 11, no. 9 (2011): 895–903. doi:10.1016/j.spinee.2011.08.006.

25 Lorimer Moseley, "Combined Physiotherapy and Education is Efficacious for Chronic Low Back Pain," *Australian J Physiotherapy* 48, no. 4 (2002): 297-302.

Chapter 6- Today's Medical Business

26 Peter Ubel, "Is The Profit Motive Ruining American Healthcare?" last modified on February 12, 2014, http://www.forbes.com/sites/peterubel/2014/02/12/is-the-profit-motive-ruining-american-healthcare/.

27 Richard A. Deyo, *Watch Your Back: How the Back Pain Industry is Costing Us More and Giving Us Less* (Ithaca and London: Cornell University Press, 2014).

28 "Health Insurance CEO Pay Sky-Rockets in 2013," last modified May 5, 2014, http://www.prnewswire.com/news-releases/health-insurance-ceo-pay-sky-rockets-in-2013-257974651.html.

Chapter 7- Different Approaches in Medicine

29 National Cancer Institute, accessed on March 7, 2015. http://www.cancer.gov/dictionary?cdrid=449752.

30 Association of American Medical Colleges, accessed on May 19, 2015. https://www.aamc.org/about/membership/378788/medicalschools.html.

31 American Association of Colleges of Osteopathic Medicine, accessed on May 19, 2015. http://www.aacom.org/become-a-doctor/about-om/US-vs-abroad.

32 American Osteopathic Association, accessed on March 7, 2015. http://www.osteopathic.org/inside-aoa/about/leadership/Pages/tenets-of-osteopathic-medicine.aspx.

33 Consortium of Academic Health Centers for Integrative Medicine, accessed March 7, 2015. http://www.imconsortium.org/about/.

Chapter 8- The Opioid Fiasco

34 Roger Chou et al, "The Effectiveness and Risks of Long-Term Opioid Therapy for Chronic Pain: A Systematic Review for a National Institutes of Health Pathways to Prevention Workshop," *Annals of Internal Medicine* 162, no. 4 (2015): 276-86. doi:10.7326/M14-2559.

35 David B. Reuben et al, "National Institutes of Health Pathways to Prevention Workshop: The Role of Opioids in the Treatment of Chronic Pain," *Annals of Internal Medicine* 163, no. 4 (2015): 295-300. doi:10.7326/M14-2775.

36 Robert Schleip et al, *Fascia: The Tensional Network of The Human Body* (London: Churchill Livingstone Elsevier, 2012), 152.

37 William M. Thomson et al, "Xerostomia and Medications among 32-year-olds," *Acta Odontologica Scandinavica* 64, no. 4 (2006): 249–54.

38 A. Baldini, Michael V. Korff, and Elizabeth H.B. Lin, "A Review of Potential Adverse Effects of Long-Term Opioid Therapy: A Practitioner's Guide," *Prim Care Companion CNS Disord* 14, no. 3 (2012): PCC.11m01326. doi:10.4088/PCC.11m01326.

39 Lucy Chen et al, "Clinical Interpretation of Opioid Tolerance versus Opioid-Induced Hyperalgesia," *J Opioid Management* 10, no. 6 (2014): 383-93. doi:10.5055/jom.2014.0235.

40 Jarred W. Younger et al, "Prescription Opioid Analgesics Rapidly Change the Human Brain," *Pain* 152, no. 8 (2011): 1803-10. doi:10.1016/j.pain.2011.03.028.

41 Matthew Miller et al, "Prescription Opioid Duration of Action and the Risk of Unintentional Overdose Among Patients Receiving Opioid Therapy," *JAMA Internal Medicine.* [Published online February 16, 2015] doi: 10.1001/jamainternmed.2014.8071.

42 Laxmaiah Manchikanti et al, "Therapeutic Use, Abuse, and Nonmedical Use of Opioids: A Ten-Year Perspective, *Pain Physician* 13 (2010): 401-35.

43 Laxmaiah Manchikanti and Angelie Singh, "Therapeutic Opioids: A Ten-Year Perspective on the Complexities and Complications of the Escalating Use, Abuse, and Nonmedical Use of Opioids," *Pain Physician* 11, suppl. 2 (2008): S63-S88.

44 Andrew Kolodny et al, "The Prescription Opioid and Heroin Crisis: A Public Health Approach to an Epidemic of Addiction," *Annual Review of Public Health* 36 [Published online January 12, 2015]: 559-574. doi:10.1146/annurev-publhealth-031914-122957.

45 Russell K. Portenoy, "Opioid Therapy for Chronic Nonmalignant Pain: Clinicians' Perspective," *J Law, Medicine & Ethics* 24 (1996): 296–309.

46 Russell K. Portenoy and Kathleen M. Foley, "Chronic Use of Opioid Analgesics in Non-Malignant Pain: Report of 38 Cases," *Pain* 25, no. 2 (1986): 171–86. doi:10.1016/0304-3959(86)90091-6.

47 Jane Porter and Hershel Jick, "Addiction Rare in Patients Treated with Narcotics," *New England J Medicine* 302, no. 2 (1980): 123.

48 Barry Meier, "In Guilty Plea, OxyContin Maker to Pay $600 Million," *New York Times*, accessed on March 7, 2015, http://www.nytimes.com/2007/05/10/business/11drug-web.html?_r=0.

49 "Opioids Drive Continued Increase in Drug Overdose Deaths," accessed January 15, 2015. http://www.cdc.gov/media/releases/2013/p0220_drug_overdose_deaths.html.

50 David Dolinak, "The Large Role of Prescription Drugs in Accidental Drug Deaths," *Academic Forensic Pathology* 3, No. 2 (2013): 222-30.

51 "Opioid Painkiller Prescribing," accessed March 22, 2015, http://www.cdc.gov/vitalsigns/opioid-prescribing/.

52 Corey S. Davis et al, "Expanded Access to Naloxone Among Firefighters, Police Officers, and Emergency Medical Technicians in Massachusetts," *American J Public Health* 104, No. 8 (2014): e7–9. doi:10.2105/AJPH.2014.302062.

53 Anna V. Williams, John Marsden, and John Strang, "Training Family Members to Manage Heroin Overdose and Administer Naloxone: Randomized Trial of Effects on Knowledge and Attitudes," *Addiction* 109, no. 2 (2014): 250–9. doi:10.1111/add.12360.

54 Thomas Catan and Evan Perez, "A Pain-Drug Champion Has Second Thoughts," *Wall Street Journal*, last modified December 17, 2012, http://www.wsj.com/articles/SB10001424127887324478304578173342657044604.

55 "Opioids for Chronic Pain: Addiction is Not Rare," Video with Dr. Russell Portenoy's perspective, uploaded October 30, 2011, accessed March 22, 2015, https://www.youtube.com/watch?v=DgyuBWN9D4w.

56 Suzanne Nielsen et al, "Benzodiazepine Use among Chronic Pain Patients Prescribed Opioids: Associations with Pain, Physical and Mental Health, and Health Service Utilization," *Pain Med* 16, no. 2 (2015): 356-66. doi:10.1111/pme.12594.

57 Jermaine D. Jones, Shanthi Mogali, and Sandra D. Comer, "Polydrug Abuse: A Review of Opioid and Benzodiazepine Combination Use," *Drug and Alcohol Dependence* 125, No. 1-2 (2012): 8-18.

58 Stephen W. Patrick et al, "Prescription Opioid Epidemic and Infant Outcomes," *Pediatrics* (published online April 13, 2015). doi: 10.1542/peds.2014-3299.

59 Seddon R. Savage, Kenneth L. Kirsh, and Steve D. Passik, "Challenges in Using Opioids to Treat Pain in Persons With Substance Use Disorders," *Addiction Science & Clinical Practice* 4, no. 2 (2008): 4-25.

60 Gary M. Franklin, "Opioids for Chronic Noncancer Pain: A Position Paper of the American Academy of Neurology," *Neurology* 83 (2014): 1277–84. doi:10.1212/WNL.0000000000000839.

61 GoodRx, accessed January 30, 2015, www.goodrx.com.

Chapter 9- Conventional Pain Medicine Procedures

62 Eugene J. Carragee et al, "2009 ISSLS Prize Winner: Does Discography Cause Accelerated Progression of Degeneration Changes in the Lumbar Disc: A Ten-Year Matched Cohort Study," *Spine* 34, no. 21 (2009): 2338-45. doi:10.1097/BRS.0b013e3181ab5432.

63 Eugene J. Carragee, Steve J. Paragioudakis, and Sanjay Khurana, "2000 Volvo Award Winner in Clinical Studies: Lumbar High-Intensity Zone and Discography in Subjects Without Low Back Problems." *Spine* 25, no. 23 (2000): 2987-92.

64 Johannes Gossner, "The Lumbar Multifidus Muscles are Affected by Medial Branch Interventions for Facet Joint Syndrome: Potential Problems and Proposal of a Pericapsular Infiltration Technique," *American J Neuroradiology* 32, no. 11 (2011): E213. doi:10.3174/ajnr.A2901.

65 John Quintner, Geoffrey Bove, and Milton Cohen, "A Critical Evaluation of the Trigger Point Phenomenon," *Rheumatology* 54, no. 3 (2015): 392-9.

66 David Simons, Janet Travell, and Lois Simons, *Myofascial Pain and Dysfunction: The Trigger Point Manual*, 2nd ed., Vol. 1-2, (Philadelphia: Lippincott, Williams & Wilkins, 1999).

67 Po-Chou Liliang et al, "The Therapeutic Efficacy of Sacroiliac Joint Blocks with Triamcinolone Acetonide in the Treatment of Sacroiliac Joint Dysfunction Without Spondyloarthropathy," *Spine* 34, no. 9 (2009): 896-900. doi:10.1097/BRS.0b013e31819e2c78.

68 Yves Maugars et al, "Assessment of the Efficacy of Sacroiliac Corticosteroid Injections in Spondyloarthropathies: A Double-Blind Study," *British J Rheumatology* 35 (1996): 767-70.

69 Ilhan Gunaydin et al, "Magnetic Resonance Imaging Guided Corticosteroid Injection of Sacroiliac Joints in Patients with Spondyloarthropathy. Are Multiple Injections More Beneficial?" *Rheumatology International* 26, no. 5 (2006): 396-400.

70 Steven P. Cohen, "Sacroiliac Joint Pain: A Comprehensive Review of Anatomy, Diagnosis, and Treatment," *Anesthesia & Analgesia* 101, no. 5 (2005): 1440-53.

71 Steven P. Cohen, Yian Chen, and Nathan J Neufeld, "Sacroiliac Joint Pain: A Comprehensive Review of Epidemiology, Diagnosis and Treatment," *Expert Review of Neurotherapeutics* 13, no. 1 (2013): 99-116. doi:10.1586/ern.12.148.

72 Hans C. Hansen et al, "Sacroiliac Joint Interventions: A Systematic Review," *Pain Physician* 10, no. 1 (2007): 165-84.

73 Cynthia Peterson and Juerg Hodler, "Evidence-Based Radiology (Part 1): Is There Sufficient Research to Support the Use of Therapeutic Injections for the Spine and Sacroiliac Joints?" *Skeletal Radiology* 39, no. 1 (2010): 5-9. doi:10.1007/s00256-009-0783-x.

74 Craig Liebenson, "The Relationship of the Sacroiliac Joint, Stabilization Musculature, and Lumbo-Pelvic Instability," *Journal of Bodywork and Movement Therapies* 8 (2004): 43-45. doi:10.1016/S1360-8592(03)00090-1.

75 "FDA Approves Spinal Cord Stimulation System that Treats Pain without Tingling Sensation," FDA News Release (May 8, 2015), accessed

online on May 12, 2015. http://www.fda.gov/NewsEvents/Newsroom/PressAnnouncements/ucm446354.htm

76 Surgery Pricing at Surgery Center of Oklahoma, accessed on January 30, 2015. http://www.surgerycenterok.com/pricing/.

77 Jaimy Lee, "New Models Send Spinal Cord Stimulator Prices Up 8%," January 23, 2015. http://www.modernhealthcare.com/article/20150123/NEWS/301239936.

78 Rachelle Buchbinder, Margaret Staples, and Damien Jolley, "Doctors With a Special Interest in Back Pain Have Poorer Knowledge About How to Treat Back Pain," *Spine* 34, No. 11 (2009): 1218-26.

Chapter 10- The Good, The Bad, and The Ugly of Surgery

79 Robert J. Gatchel and Kathryn H. Rollings, "Evidence-Informed Management of Chronic Low Back Pain with Cognitive Behavioral Therapy," *Spine Journal* 8, no. 1 (2008): 40-44. doi:10.1016/j.spinee.2007.10.007.

80 Jason C. Eck, et al, "Guideline Update for the Performance of Fusion Procedures for Degenerative Disease of the Lumbar Spine. Part 7: Lumbar Fusion for Intractable Low-Back Pain Without Stenosis or Spondylolisthesis," *J Neurosurgery* 21, no. 1 (2014): 42–47. doi:10.3171/2014.4.SPINE14270.

81 William C. Watters III et al, "Guideline Update for the Performance of Fusion Procedures for Degenerative Disease of the Lumbar Spine. Part 13: Injection Therapies, Low-Back Pain, and Lumbar Fusion," *J Neurosurgery* 21, no. 1 (2014): 79-90.

82 Jeffrey C. Wang et al, "Guideline Update for the Performance of Fusion Procedures for Degenerative Disease of the Lumbar Spine. Part 8: Lumbar Fusion for Disc Herniation and Radiculopathy," *J Neurosurgery* 21, no. 1 (2014): 48-53.

83 Michael W. Groff et al, "Guideline Update for the Performance of Fusion Procedures for Degenerative Disease of the Lumbar Spine. Part 12: Pedicle Screw Fixation as an Adjunct to Posterolateral Fusion," *J Neurosurgery* 21, no. 1 (2014): 75-78.

84 Eugene J. Carragee, "The Role of Surgery in Low Back Pain," *Current Orthopaedics* 21 (2007): 9-16.

85 Eugene J. Carragee, "Surgical Treatment of Lumbar Disk Disorders," *J American Medical Association* 296, no. 20 (2006): 2485-87. doi:10.1001/jama.296.20.2485.

86 Roger Chou et al, "Surgery for Low Back Pain: A Review of the Evidence for an American Pain Society Clinical Practice Guideline," *Spine* 34, no. 10 (2009): 1094-1109. doi:10.1097/BRS.0b013e3181a105fc.

87 Eck et al, "Lumbar Spine. Part 7," 2014 (see note 80).

88 William J. Mixter and Joseph S. Barr, "Rupture of the Intervertebral Disc with Involvement of the Spinal Canal," *New England J Medicine* 211 (1934): 210-15. doi:10.1056/NEJM193408022110506.

89 Robert J. Gatchel and Akiko Okifuji, "Evidence-Based Scientific Data Documenting the Treatment and Cost-Effectiveness of Comprehensive Pain Programs for Chronic Nonmalignant Pain," *J Pain* 7, no. 11 (2006): 779-93. doi:10.1016/j.jpain.2006.08.005.

90 Surgery Pricing at Surgery Center of Oklahoma, accessed January 30, 2015, http://www.surgerycenterok.com/pricing/.

91 "LumbarLynne," July 25, 2009 (3:45pm), "Cost of Lumbar Fusion Surgery - $90 K," post on *Spine-health Back Surgery and Neck Surgery patient community,* accessed on January 30, 2015, http://www.spine-health.com/forum/treatment/back-surgery-and-neck-surgery/cost-lumbar-fusion-surgery-90-k.

92 J. Bruce Moseley et al, "A Controlled Trial of Arthroscopic Surgery for Osteoarthritis of the Knee," *New England J Medicine* 347 (2002): 81-88. doi:10.1056/NEJMoa013259.

93 Nicolas H von der Hoeh et al, "Impact of a Multidisciplinary Pain Program for the Management of Chronic Low Back Pain in Patients Undergoing Spine Surgery and Primary Total Hip Replacement: A Retrospective Cohort Study," *Patient Safety in Surgery* 8 (2014): 34. doi:10.1186/s13037-014-0034-5.

94 "Minimally Invasive Surgery: Continuing Mismatch Between Marketing Claims and Scientific Reality?" *The Back Letter* (Hagerstown, MD: Lippincott Williams & Wilkins monthly newsletter, 2015) 30, no. 5: 56.

Chapter 11- Limitations of Evidence-Based Medicine

95 Birger Hjørland, "Evidence-Based Practice: An Analysis Based on the Philosophy of Science," *J Association for Information Science and Technology* 62, no. 7 (2011): 1301-10. doi:10.1002/asi.21523.

96 David L. Sackett et al, "Evidence Based Medicine: What it Is and What it Isn't," *BMJ* 312 (1996): 71. doi:10.1136/bmj.312.7023.71.

97 Gordon C. S. Smith and Jill P. Pell, "Parachute Use to Prevent Death and Major Trauma Related to Gravitational Challenge: Systematic Review of Randomised Controlled Trials," *Int J Prosthodont* 19 (2006): 126-28. [Reprint from *BMJ* 327 (2003):1459-61.]

98 Trisha Greenhalgh, Jeremy Howick, and Neal Maskrey, "Evidence-Based Medicine: a Movement in Crisis?" *BMJ* 348 (2014): g3725. doi:10.1136/bmj.g3725.

99 Stefan Timmermans and Aaron Mauck, "The Promises and Pitfalls of Evidence-Based Medicine," *Health Affairs* 24, no. 1 (2005): 18–28. doi:10.1377/hlthaff.24.1.18.

Chapter 12- The Disk Risk: Understanding the *Disc*-onnect!

100 David G. Borenstein et al, "The Value of Magnetic Resonance Imaging of the Lumbar Spine to Predict Low-Back Pain in Asymptomatic Subjects: A Seven-Year Follow-Up Study," *J Bone & Joint Surgery* 83, no. 9 (2001): 1306-11.

101 Eugene J. Carragee et al, "Are First-Time Episodes of Serious LBP Associated with New MRI Findings?" *Spine Journal* 6, no. 6 (2006): 624-35. doi:10.1016/j.spinee.2006.03.005.

102 Scott D. Boden et al, "Abnormal Magnetic-Resonance Scans of the Cervical Spine in Asymptomatic Subjects. A Prospective Investigation," *J Bone & Joint Surgery* 72, no. 8 (1990): 1178-84.

103 Roger Chou et al, "Imaging Strategies for Low-Back Pain: Systematic Review and Meta-Analysis," *Lancet* 373, no. 9662 (2009): 463-72. doi:10.1016/S0140-6736(09)60172-0.

104 Waleed Brinjikji et al, "Systematic Literature Review of Imaging Features of Spinal Degeneration in Asymptomatic Populations," *American J Neuroradiology* [Published online on November 27, 2014]. doi:10.3174/ajnr.A4173.

105 Robert Dallek, *An Unfinished Life: John F. Kennedy, 1917-1963* (New York: Back Bay Books, 2013).

106 Ibid, 694.

Chapter 13- Are you *Diagnocentric*™?

107 Ray Moynihan, Jenny Doust, and David Henry, "Preventing Overdiagnosis: How to Stop Harming the Healthy," *BMJ 344 (*2012): e3502. doi:10.1136/bmj.e3502.

Chapter 14- The Pain Patient Funnel

108 Vincent Scaia, David Baxter, and Chad Cook, "The Pain Provocation-Based Straight Leg Raise Test for Diagnosis of Lumbar Disc Herniation, Lumbar Radiculopathy, and/or Sciatica: A Systematic Review of Clinical Utility," *J Back and Musculoskeletal Rehabilitation* 25, no. 4 (2012): 215-23. doi:10.3233/BMR-2012-0339.

109 Richard A. Deyo et al, "Overtreating Chronic Back Pain: Time to Back Off?" *J American Board of Family Medicine* 22, no. 1 (2009): 62–68. doi:10.3122/jabfm.2009.01.080102.

Chapter 15- Bridging a Gap: Biomechanics

110 OP VK Project, "Biomechanical basis for Physical Exercises," accessed online on March 7, 2015, http://www.fsps.muni.cz/~tvodicka/data/reader/book-2/02.html.

111 Sanne T. Christensen and Jan Hartvigsen, "Spinal Curves and Health: A Systematic Critical Review of Epidemiological Literature Dealing with

Associations Between Sagittal Spinal Curves and Health," *J Manipulative Physiological Therapeutics* 31, no. 9 (2008): 690-714. doi:10.1016/j.jmpt.2008.10.004.

112 Personal communication and lecture by Stuart McGill, Winnipeg, Canada, April 12, 2015.

113 Ibid.

Chapter 16- A Missing Link: Connective Tissue

114 Schleip, *Fascia,* xvii (see Chapter 8, note 36).

115 Zeynep Firtina et al, "Abnormal Expression of Collagen IV in Lens Activates Unfolded Protein Response Resulting in Cataract," *J Biological Chemistry* 284 (2009): 35872-84. doi:10.1074/jbc.M109.060384.

116 Jean-Claude Guimberteau, "Strolling Under The Skin," Video produced by EndoVivo Productions, 2005.

117 Helene M. Langevin, "The Science of Stretch." *The Scientist,* last modified May 1, 2013, http://www.the-scientist.com/?articles.view/articleNo/35301/title/The-Science-of-Stretch/.

118 Ibid.

119 Helene M. Langevin et al, "Dynamic Fibroblast Cytoskeletal Response to Subcutaneous Tissue Stretch Ex Vivo and In Vivo," *American J Physiology - Cell Physiology* 288 (2005): C747–56. doi:10.1152/ajpcell.00420.2004.

120 Helene M. Langevin et al, "Ultrasound Evidence of Altered Lumbar Connective Tissue Structure in Human Subjects with Chronic Low Back Pain," *BMC Musculoskeletal Disorders* 151 (2009): published online. doi:10.1186/1471-2474-10-151.

121 Helene M. Langevin et al, "Reduced Thoracolumbar Fascia Shear Strain in Human Chronic Low Back Pain," *BMC Musculoskeletal Disorders* 203 (2011): published online. doi:10.1186/1471-2474-12-203.

122 Sarah M. Corey et al, "Sensory Innervation of the Nonspecialized Connective Tissues in the Low Back of the Rat," *Cells Tissues Organs* 194 (2011): 521–30. doi:10.1159/000323875.

123 Lemont H, Ammirati K, and Usen N, "Plantar fasciitis: a degenerative process (fasciosis) without inflammation." *J American Podiatric Medical Association* 93, no. 3 (2003): 234-37.

124 Raymond R. Monto, "Platelet-Rich Plasma Efficacy Versus Corticosteroid Injection Treatment for Chronic Severe Plantar Fasciitis," *Foot Ankle Intern* 35, no. 4 (2014): 313-18. doi: 10.1177/1071100713519778.

125 Langevin, "Dynamic Fibroblast," (see note 119).

126 Helene M. Langevin et al, "Fibroblast Cytoskeletal Remodeling Contributes to Connective Tissue Tension," *J Cellular Physiology* 226, no. 5 (2011): 1166-75. doi:10.1002/jcp.22442.

127 Helene M. Langevin et al, "Fibroblast Cytoskeletal Remodeling Induced by Tissue Stretch Involves ATP Signaling," *J Cellular Physiology* 228, no. 9 (2013): 1922-6. doi:10.1002/jcp.24356.

128 Corey, "Sensory Innervation," (see note 122).

129 Toshiyuki Saito et al, "Analysis of the Posterior Ramus of the Lumbar Spinal Nerve: The Structure of the Posterior Ramus of the Spinal Nerve," *J Amer Society of Anesthesiologists* 118 (2013): 88-94. doi:10.1097/ALN.0b013e318272f40a.

130 *The Management of Pain*, 2nd edition, ed. by John J. Bonica, with John D. Loeser, C. Richard Chapman, and Wilbert E. Fordyce (Philadelphia: Lea and Febiger, 1990): 139-140.

Chapter 17- No Brain, No Pain: The Nervous System

131 Helene M. Langevin and Karen J. Sherman, "Pathophysiological Model For Chronic Low Back Pain Integrating Connective Tissue and Nervous System Mechanisms," *Medical Hypotheses* 68, no. 1 (2006): 74-80. doi:10.1016/j.mehy.2006.06.033.

132 Doidge, *The Brain*, 177-195, (see Chapter 1, note 5).

133 Lidia Bravo et al, "Depressive-Like States Heighten the Aversion to Painful Stimuli in a Rat Model of Comorbid Chronic Pain and Depression," *Anesthesiology* 117, no. 3 (2012): 613-25. doi:10.1097/ALN.0b013e3182657b3e.

134 Jarred Younger et al, "Viewing Pictures of a Romantic Partner Reduces Experimental Pain: Involvement of Neural Reward Systems," *PLoS ONE* 5, no. 10 (2010): e13309. doi:10.1371/journal.pone.0013309.

135 Ibid.

136 Jonathan Greenberg, Keren Reiner, and Nachshon Meiran, "Off with the old: mindfulness practice improves backward inhibition," *Frontiers in Psychology* 3 (2013): Article 618. doi:10.3389/fpsyg.2012.00618.

137 Bram P. Prins, A. Decuypere, and Stefaan Van Damme, "Effects of Mindfulness and Distraction on Pain Depend upon Individual Differences in Pain Catastrophizing: An Experimental Study," *European J Pain* 18, no. 9 (2014): 1307-15. doi:10.1002/j.1532-2149.2014.491.x.

138 Beth Darnall, *Less Pain, Fewer Pills: Avoid the Dangers of Prescription Opioids and Gain Control over Chronic Pain* (Boulder, Colorado: Bull Publishing Company, 2014).

139 Ruth Defrin et al, "The Long-Term Impact of Tissue Injury on Pain Processing and Modulation: A Study on Ex-Prisoners of War Who Underwent Torture," *European J Pain* 18, no. 4 (2014): 548-58. doi:10.1002/j.1532-2149.2013.00394.x.

140 R.H. Gracely et al, "Pain Catastrophizing and Neural Responses to Pain Among Persons with Fibromyalgia," *Brain* 127 (2004): 835-43. doi:10.1093/brain/awh098.

141 David A. Seminowicz and Karen D. Davis, "Cortical Responses to Pain in Healthy Individuals Depends on Pain Catastrophizing," *Pain* 120 (2006): 297–306. doi:10.1016/j.pain.2005.11.008.

142 Susan J. Picavet, Johan W. S. Vlaeyen, and Jan S. A. G. Schouten, "Pain Catastrophizing and Kinesiophobia: Predictors of Chronic Low Back Pain," *American J Epidemiology* 156, no. 11 (2002): 1028–34. doi:10.1093/aje/kwf136.

143 Jeroen de Jong, et al, "Fear of Movement/(Re)injury in Chronic Low Back Pain: Education or Exposure In Vivo as Mediator to Fear Reduction?" *Clinical J Pain* 21, no. 1 (2005): 9-17. doi:10.1097/00002508-200501000-00002.

144 Ilse Swinkels-Meewisse et al, "Acute Low Back Pain: Pain-Related Fear and Pain Catastrophizing Influence Physical Performance and Perceived Disability," *Pain* 120 (2006): 36–43. doi:10.1016/j.pain.2005.10.005.

145 G. Lorimer Moseley, "Evidence for a Direct Relationship Between Cognitive and Physical Change During an Education Intervention in People with Chronic Low Back Pain," *European J Pain* 8, no. 1 (2004): 39-45. doi:10.1016/S1090-3801(03)00063-6.

146 G. Lorimer Moseley, "Combined Physiotherapy and Education is Efficacious for Chronic Low Back Pain," *Australian J Physiotherapy* 48, no. 4 (2002): 297-302.

147 G. Lorimer Moseley, "Joining Forces—Combining Cognition-Targeted Motor Control Training with Group or Individual Pain Physiology Education: A Successful Treatment for Chronic Low Back Pain," *J Manual and Manipulative Therapy* 11, no. 2 (2003): 88-94.

148 Robert J. Brison et al, "A Randomized Controlled Trial of an Educational Intervention to Prevent the Chronic Pain of Whiplash Associated Disorders Following Rear-End Motor Vehicle Collisions," *Spine* 30, no. 16 (2005): 1799-1807.

149 Mimi Mehlsen, Lea Heegaard, and Lisbeth Frostholm, "A Prospective Evaluation of the Chronic Pain Self-Management Programme in a Danish Population of Chronic Pain Patients," *Patient Education and Counseling.* [Published online January 19, 2015]. doi: 10.1016/j.pec.2015.01.008.

150 A. Vanhaudenhuyse et al, "Efficacy and Cost-Effectiveness: A Study of Different Treatment Approaches in a Tertiary Pain Centre," *European J Pain* [Published online February 24, 2015]. doi: 10.1002/ejp.674.

151 Neil Pearson, personal communication with author, March 16, 2015.

Chapter 19- Know Your "Home": Pay Attention To Your Body

152 Aging Definition, National Institutes of Health, accessed March 22, 2015, http://www.nlm.nih.gov/medlineplus/ency/article/004012.htm.

153 Kenneth Minaker, "Common Clinical Sequelae of Aging," in *Goldman's Cecil Medicine*, 24th ed., ed. Lee Goldman (Philadelphia, PA: Elsevier Saunders, 2011), chap. 24.

154 P. Zimmer and W. Block, "Physical Exercise and Epigenetic Adaptations of the Cardiovascular System," *Herz* [Published online March 7, 2015].

155 Malgorzata Wegner et al, "Role of epigenetic mechanisms in the development of chronic complications of diabetes," *Diabetes Research and Clinical Practice* 105, no. 2 (2014): 164-75. doi:10.1016/j.diabres.2014.03.019.

156 Darrell L. Ellsworth et al, "Intensive Cardiovascular Risk Reduction Induces Sustainable Changes in Expression of Genes and Pathways Important to Vascular Function," *Circulation: Cardiovascular Genetics* 7, no. 2 (2014): 151–60. doi:10.1161/CIRCGENETICS.113.000121.

157 Bi-Kui Zhang, Xin Lai, and Sujie Jia, "Epigenetics in Atherosclerosis: A Clinical Perspective," *Discovery Medicine*. [Published online on February 19, 2015]: 74-80. http://www.discoverymedicine.com/Bi-Kui-Zhang/2015/02/epigenetics-in-atherosclerosis-a-clinical-perspective/.

158 Gordon Waddell, "Volvo Award in Clinical Sciences. A New Clinical Model for the Treatment of Low-Back Pain," *Spine* 12, no. 7 (1987): 632-44.

159 Astrid Bjornebekk, Aleksander A. Mathe, and Stefan Brene, "The Antidepressant Effect of Running is Associated with Increased Hippocampal Cell Proliferation," *International J Neuropsychopharmacology* 8, no. 3 (2005): 357-68. doi:10.1017/S1461145705005122.

160 Matthew D. Jones et al, "Aerobic Training Increases Pain Tolerance in Healthy Individuals," *Medicine & Science in Sports & Exercise* 46, no. 8 (2014): 1640-47. doi:10.1249/MSS.0000000000000273.

161 Deirdre A. Hurley et al, "Supervised Walking in Comparison with Fitness Training for Chronic Back Pain in Physiotherapy: Results of the SWIFT Single-Blinded Randomized Controlled Trial," *Pain* 156, no. 1 (2015): 131-147. doi:10.1016/j.pain.0000000000000013.

162 Ulrich John et al, "Tobacco Smoking in Relation to Pain in a National General Population Survey," *Preventive Medicine* 43, no. 6 (2006): 477–81. doi:10.1016/j.ypmed.2006.07.005.

163 Molly T. Vogt et al, "Influence of Smoking on the Health Status of Spinal Patients: The National Spine Network Database," *Spine* 27, no. 3 (2002): 313–19.

164 Jenna Goesling, Chad M. Brummett and Afton L. Hassett, "Cigarette Smoking and Pain: Depression Symptoms Mediate Smoking-Related Pain Symptoms," *Pain* 153, no. 8 (2012): 1749-54.

165 M.C. Battié et al, "1991 Volvo Award in Clinical Sciences. Smoking and Lumbar Intervertebral Disc Degeneration: An MRI Study of Identical Twins," *Spine* 16, no. 9 (1991): 1015-21.

166 Caleb Behrend et al, "Smoking Cessation Related to Improved Patient-Reported Pain Scores Following Spinal Care," *J Bone Joint Surgery* 94, no. 23 (2012): 2161-66. doi:10.2106/JBJS.K.01598.

167 Robert N. Proctor, *Golden Holocaust: Origins of the Cigarette Catastrophe and the Case for Abolition* (Berkeley and Los Angeles, California: University of California Press, 2012).

168 Ola Ekholm et al, "Alcohol and Smoking Behavior in Chronic Pain Patients: The Role of Opioids," *European J Pain* 13, no. 6 (2009): 606-12. doi:10.1016/j.ejpain.2008.07.006.

169 Bogdan Petre et al, "Smoking Increases Risk of Pain Chronification Through Shared Corticostriatal Circuitry," *Human Brain Mapping* 36, no. 2 (2015): 683-94. doi:10.1002/hbm.22656.

170 Institute of Medicine, "Dietary Reference Intakes for Water, Potassium, Sodium, Chloride, and Sulfate," last modified 2004, accessed March 22, 2015, http://www.iom.edu/Global/News%20Announcements/~/media/442A08B899F44DF9AAD083D86164C75B.ashx.

171 Neal D. Barnard, *Foods That Fight Pain* (United States: Rodale Publishing, 2008), 214.

172 Mark Hyman, MD, "Milk is Dangerous for Your Health," accessed March 7, 2015, http://drhyman.com/blog/2013/10/28/milk-dangerous-health/.

173 Diane Feskanich, Walter C. Willett and Graham A. Colditz, "Calcium, Vitamin D, Milk Consumption, and Hip Fractures: A Prospective Study Among Postmenopausal Women," *American Society for Clinical Nutrition* 77, no. 2 (2003): 504-11.

174 Barnard, *Foods*, 14 (see note 171).

175 Deborah E. Sellmeyer et al, "A High Ratio of Dietary Animal to Vegetable Protein Increases the Rate of Bone Loss and the Risk of Fracture in Postmenopausal Women," *American J Clinical Nutrition* 73, no. 1 (2001): 118-22.

176 David S. Ludwig and Walter C. Willett, "Three Daily Servings of Reduced-Fat Milk: An Evidence-Based Recommendation?" *JAMA Pediatrics* 167, no. 9 (2013): 788-89. doi:10.1001/jamapediatrics.2013.2408.

177 Gert Hein and S. Franke, "Are Advanced Glycation End-Product-Modified Proteins of Pathogenetic Importance in Fibromyalgia?" *Rheumatology* 41, no. 10 (2002): 1163-67. doi:10.1093/rheumatology/41.10.1163.

178 Barnard, *Foods*, 82-85 (see note 171).

179 L.I. Kauppila, "Atherosclerosis and Disc Degeneration/Low-Back Pain – A Systematic Review," *European J Vascular & Endovascular Surgery* 37, no. 6 (2009): 661-70. doi:10.1016/j.ejvs.2009.02.006.

180 John L. Doppman and Giovanni Di Chiro, "Paraspinal Muscle Infarction. A Painful Complication of Lumbar Artery Embolization Associated with Pathognomonic Radiographic and Laboratory Findings," *Radiology* 119, no. 3 (1976): 609-13. doi:10.1148/119.3.609.

181 Phillip Tuso, Scott R. Stoll, and William W Li, "A Plant-Based Diet, Atherogenesis, and Coronary Artery Disease Prevention," *Permanente Journal* 19, no. 1 (2015): 62-67. doi:10.7812/TPP/14-036.

182 Richard A. Deyo and JE Bass, "Lifestyle and Low-Back Pain: The Influence of Smoking and Obesity," *Spine* 14, no. 5 (1989): 501-6.

183 Barnard, *Foods* (see note 171).

184 Jeon Younghoon et al, "Curcumin Could Prevent the Development of Chronic Neuropathic Pain in Rats with Peripheral Nerve Injury," *Curr Therapeutic Research* 74 (2013): 1-4.

185 Melissa S. Monsey et al, "A Diet Enriched with Curcumin Impairs Newly Acquired and Reactivated Fear Memories," *Neuropsychopharmacology* 13, no. 40 (2015): 1278-88. doi:10.1038/npp.2014.315.

186 Mary Norval and H.C. Wulf, "Does Chronic Sunscreen Use Reduce Vitamin D Production to Insufficient Levels?" *British J Dermatology* 161, no. 4 (2009): 732-36. doi:10.1111/j.1365-2133.2009.09332.x.

187 John McBeth, Rosie J. Lacey, and Ross Wilkie, "Predictors of New Onset Widespread Pain in Older Adults: Results from a Population-Based Prospective Cohort Study in the UK," *Arthritis & Rheumatology* 66, no. 3 (2014): 757-67. doi:10.1002/art.38284.

188 T. Roehrs et al, "Sleep Loss and REM Sleep Loss are Hyperalgesic," *Sleep* 29, no. 2 (2006): 145-151.

189 Sigrid Schuh-Hofer et al, "One Night of Total Sleep Deprivation Promotes a State of Generalized Hyperalgesia: A Surrogate Pain Model to Study the Relationship of Insomnia and Pain," *Pain* 154, no. 9 (2013): 1613-21. doi:10.1016/j.pain.2013.04.046.

190 Joel E. Dimsdale et al, "The Effect of Opioids on Sleep Architecture," *J Clinical Sleep Medicine,* 3, no. 1 (2007): 33-36.

191 Julia K.M. Chan et al, "The Acute Effects of Alcohol on Sleep Electroencephalogram Power Spectra in Late Adolescence," *Alcoholism: Clinical and Experimental Research* 39, no. 2 (2015): 291-99. doi:10.1111/acer.12621.

192 Arthur A. Stone and Joan E. Broderick, "Obesity and Pain Are Associated in the United States," *Obesity* 20, no. 7 (2012): 1-5. doi:10.1038/oby.2011.397.

193 Jarred Younger et al, "Viewing Pictures of a Romantic Partner Reduces Experimental Pain: Involvement of Neural Reward Systems," PLoS ONE 5, no. 10 (2010): e13309. doi:10.1371/journal.pone.0013309.

194 Neil Pearson, personal communication with author, March 16, 2015.

195 Neil Pearson, email communication with author, March 22, 2015.

196 David H. Bradshaw et al, "Individual Differences in the Effects of Music Engagement on Responses to Painful Stimulation," *J Pain* 12, no. 12 (2011): 1262-73. doi:10.1016/j.jpain.2011.08.010

197 David S. Black et al, "Mindfulness Meditation and Improvement in Sleep Quality and Daytime Impairment Among Older Adults With Sleep Disturbances: A Randomized Clinical Trial," *JAMA Intern Medicine* [Published online February 16, 2015]: E1-8. doi:10.001/jamainternmed.2014.8081.

198 Sara W. Lazar et al, "Meditation Experience is Associated with Increased Cortical Thickness," *Neuroreport* 16, no. 17 (2005): 1893-97.

199 R. Padmanabhan, A.J. Hildreth, and D. Laws, "A Prospective, Randomised, Controlled Study Examining Binaural Beat Audio and Pre-Operative Anxiety in Patients Undergoing General Anaesthesia for Day Case Surgery," *Anaesthesia* 60, no. 9 (2005): 874-77. doi:10.1111/j.1365-2044.2005.04287.x.

200 Darnall, *Less Pain*, (see Chapter 17, note 138).

201 Stelian A. Balan et al, "A Comparative Study Regarding The Efficiency Of Applying Hypnotherapeutic Techniques and Binaural Beats in Modifying the Level of Perceived Pain," *Romanian J Cognitive Behavioral Therapy and Hypnosis* 1, no. 2 (2014): 1-9.

202 Joachim Stoeber and Dirk P. Janssen, "Perfectionism and Coping with Daily Failures: Positive Reframing Helps Achieve Satisfaction at the End of the Day," *Anxiety, Stress, & Coping* 24 no. 5 (2011): 477-97. doi:10.1080/10615806.2011.562977.

203 William S. Marras et al, "The Influence of Psychosocial Stress, Gender, and Personality on Mechanical Loading of the Lumbar Spine," *Biomechanics* 25, no. 23 (2000): 3045-54.

204 Mimi M.Y. Tse, "Humor Therapy: Relieving Chronic Pain and Enhancing Happiness for Older Adults," *J Aging Research* 2010 (2010): 9 pages. doi:10.4061/2010/343574.

205 Tara L. Kraft and Sarah D. Pressman, "Grin and Bear It: The Influence of Manipulated Positive Facial Expression on the Stress

Response," *Psychological Science* 23, no. 11 (2012): 1372-78. doi:10.1177/0956797612445312.

Chapter 20- Do-It-Yourself Pain Management

206 Anava A. Wren et al, "Yoga for Persistent Pain: New Findings and Directions for an Ancient Practice," *Pain* 152, no. 3 (2011): 477-80.

207 Padmini Tekur et al, "Effect of Short-Term Intensive Yoga Program on Pain, Functional Disability and Spinal Flexibility in Chronic Low Back Pain: A Randomized Control Study," *J Altern Complement Med* 14, no. 6 (2008): 637-44. doi:10.1089/acm.2007.0815.

208 Paul Little et al, "Randomised Controlled Trial of Alexander Technique Lessons, Exercise, and Massage for Chronic and Recurrent Back Pain," *BMJ* 337 (2015): a884. doi:10.1136/bmj.a884.

209 Jean Krampe et al, "Does Dance-Based Therapy Increase Gait Speed in Older Adults with Chronic Lower Extremity Pain: A Feasibility Study," *Geriatric Nursing* 35, no. 5 (2014): 339-44. doi:10.1016/j.gerinurse.2014.03.008.

Chapter 21- Who are Your Body and Brain Assistants?

210 John C. Licciardone et al, "Osteopathic Manual Treatment and Ultrasound Therapy for Chronic Low Back Pain: A Randomized Controlled Trial," *Ann Fam* Med 11, no. 2 (2013):122-9. doi:10.1370/afm.1468.

211 John C. Licciardone, Angela K. Brimhall, and Linda N. King, "Osteopathic Manipulative Treatment for Low Back Pain: A Systematic Review and Meta-Analysis of Randomized Controlled Trials," *BMC Musculoskeletal Disorders* 6, no. 43 (2005): 12 pages. doi:10.1186/1471-2474-6-43.

212 Robert A. Leach, *The Chiropractic Theories: A Textbook of Scientific Research*, 4th ed. (New York: Lippincott, Williams and Wilkins, 2003), 15.

213 Ibid.

214 A.J. Terrett, "The Genius of D.D. Palmer: An Exploration of the Origin of Chiropractic in His Time," *Chiro History* 11, no. 1 (1991): 31-8.

215 Martin Seligman, *Learned Optimism: How to Change Your Mind and Your Life* (New York: Vintage, Reprint Edition, 2006).

Glossary

Addiction: A disease state typically characterized by behaviors that include one or more of the following: impaired control over drug use, compulsive use, continued use despite harm, and craving. Genetic, psychosocial, and environmental factors can influence its development.

Algorithm: A step-by-step protocol, such as for the management of a medical problem.

Allodynia: Condition in which ordinarily non-painful stimuli evoke pain.

Analgesia: The inability to feel pain or pain relief.

***antiPAIN Lifestyle*:** (*Term used by the author*) **The lifestyle based upon the principles of self-care using healthy challenges and choices which naturally improve quality of life and minimize pain.** By honoring a miraculous body and accepting pain's complexity, the medical community would be used as a source of education and guidance to facilitate good function with conservative treatments and occasional bridges (medications, injections, surgeries) that minimize risk and maximize benefit.

Arachnoiditis: A challenging and complex pain disorder related to inflammation of the arachnoid membrane, which surrounds the spinal nerves. Irritation can be from mechanical, infectious, chemical, or post-surgical causes.

Sometimes scar tissue develops and causes nerves to "stick together." The symptoms can range widely and unpredictably from tingling, numbness, bowel issues, bladder issues, sexual dysfunction, or paralysis. Treatment is still somewhat experimental with injections and spinal cord stimulators, etc.

Aspirate: Inspiratory sucking into the airways of fluid or foreign body, as of vomitus.

Ativan®: Brand name for lorazepam. *See Benzodiazepine.*

Benzodiazepine: Parent compound for the synthesis of a number of psychoactive compounds, such as diazepam (aka Valium) or alprazolam (aka Xanax), which can lead to side effects, such as respiratory depression and memory loss.

Biopsychosocial: Involving the interplay of biological, psychological and social influences.

Botox®: Brand name for botulin toxin. *See Botulin/Botulinus toxin.*

Botulin/Botulinus toxin: Commonly known by a brand name, Botox®. A potent neurotoxin from *Clostridium botulinum.* In large doses, it can be lethal, but in small doses some types (e.g., Type A) can be used to treat pain related to muscle spasms or cosmetically minimize wrinkles.

***Br-ody*™:** (*Term used by the author)* Term used to emphasize that the brain and body are not separate entities, but rather a complete body system. This portmanteau or blend word stems from brain + body = br-ody (pron. "braw-dee").

Catastrophizing: To view or talk about a situation or pain as worse than it actually is, or as if it were a catastrophe. To overly fixate on a problem.

Central pain: "A neurological condition caused by damage to or dysfunction of the central nervous system, which includes the brain, brainstem, and spinal cord. This syndrome can be caused by stroke, multiple sclerosis, tumors, epilepsy, brain or spinal cord trauma, or Parkinson's disease. The character of the pain associated with this syndrome differs widely among individuals partly because of the variety of potential causes. Central pain syndrome may affect a large portion of the body or may be more restricted to specific areas, such as hands or feet. The extent of pain is usually related to the cause of the CNS injury or damage. Pain is typically constant, may be moderate to severe in intensity, and is often made worse by touch, movement, emotions, and temperature changes, usually cold temperatures. Individuals experience one or more types of pain sensations, the most prominent being burning. Mingled with the burning may be sensations of "pins and needles;" pressing, lacerating, or aching pain; and brief, intolerable bursts of sharp pain similar to the pain caused by a dental probe on an exposed nerve. Individuals may have numbness in the areas affected by the pain. The burning and loss of touch sensations are usually most severe on the distant parts of the body, such as the feet or hands. Central pain syndrome often begins shortly after the causative injury or damage, but may be delayed by months or even years, especially if it is related to post-stroke pain." (*from the National Institute of Neurological Disorders and Stroke*). *See Central sensitization.*

Central sensitization/Centralization/Centralized pain/Central pain syndrome: All of these terms are interchangeable with *central pain* or *sensitization* if referring to the fact that a peripheral or central injury or disorder is creating a state of *central nervous system* over-activation and inflammation, metabolic disturbances, cellular destruction, and nerve sensitization. There is suggestion that special nervous system cells, called *glial cells*, are an integral part of this dysfunctional process. It is now appreciated that *peripheral* nerve issues can *centralize* to the brain and spinal cord. This constantly painful condition can severely impair a patient's sleep and function. Fatigue and depression can be so profound that the patient becomes reclusive and antisocial.

Chemoablation: Destruction of a body part, such as a nerve, by a chemical.

Cognitive Behavioral Therapy (CBT): A form of treatment that incorporates multiple methods such as enhancing one's awareness of thoughts, instilling motivational self-talk, minimizing self-defeating thought, or changing maladaptive beliefs about pain in order to help minimize the intensity of pain. Addressing fear-avoidance behaviors is part of this therapy. Thoughts, feeling and behaviors are the focus. Evidence suggests that the brain can improve its functioning by engaging in this type of therapy. Helpful for multiple issues including depression and anxiety, which can be a contributor or a consequence of pain.

Coinsurance: The shared expense of a medical service with the insurance company per the company's policy, but typically after the deductible is met. For example, if there is a $3,000 yearly deductible and 20% coinsurance, then the patient at best would get only 80% of a service covered *if* the $3,000 was already paid for that year.

Copay (aka copayment): A fixed payment by an insured person each time a medical service is received, if the service is covered by an insurance policy (in the United States).

Cryoablation: Destruction of a body part, such as a nerve, by freezing.

Deductible: The amount of money the patient must pay before the insurance company will cover any health care services.

Degenerative disc disease (DDD): Degeneration of intervertebral discs within the spine. Commonly seen in people with or without pain.

Dependence, Opioid: A pattern of behavioral, physiologic, and cognitive symptoms that develop due to opioid use or abuse; usually indicated by tolerance to the effects of the opioid. As a consequence, withdrawal symptoms develop when use of the substance is terminated too quickly.

Dermatome: The area of the skin supplied by the most distant (or cutaneous) branches from a single spinal nerve; neighboring dermatomes may overlap.

***Diagnocentric*™:** (*Term used by the author*) Thinking of one's self as a diagnosis, without regard to the cause of the labeled condition and without effort to change the lifestyle that may lead to or worsen that condition.

***Diagnocentricity*®:** (*Term used by the author*) The state of thinking of one's self as a diagnosis, without regard to the cause of the labeled medical condition and without effort to change the lifestyle that may lead to or worsen that condition

Disc, Intervertebral: A disk (disc) between the bodies of adjacent vertebrae. It is composed of an outer fibrous part (annulus fibrosus) that surrounds a central gelatinous mass (nucleus pulposus).

D.O.: *See Osteopathic Physician.*

Dysesthesia: An unpleasant sensation, which may or may not be painful.

Ehler's Danlos Syndromes (EDS): Related to a genetic defect in connective tissues, which results in faulty or reduced amounts of collagen leading to less strength in the tissue. EDS is a heterogeneous group of heritable connective tissue disorders characterized by articular (joint) hypermobility, skin extensibility, and tissue fragility. (*from www.ednf.org*)

Electromyography (EMG): The recording of electrical activity generated in muscle for diagnostic purposes; surface or needle electrodes can be used. *See Nerve Conduction Study.*

Epigenetics or epigenesis: Regulation of the expression of gene activity without alteration of the genetic structure or code.

Facet (zygapophyseal) joints: Synovial joints on each side of the vertebra that connect to another vertebra above or below it, allowing freedom of motion at that junction.

Failed back syndrome: A condition characterized by persistent back and/or leg pain following back surgeries. *Also known as Post-Laminectomy Syndrome.*

Fluoroscopy: A form of X-ray that can be seen on a monitor and used to take snapshots or continuous images during a procedure. Radiation exposure of varying degrees is inevitable when patients undergo pain procedures requiring fluoroscopy.

Foramen: An opening or passage, within or related to a bone. As an example, when one vertebra is stacked on top of another, a foramen is created between the two bones. The foramen allows a spinal nerve root to exit.

Foramina: Plural of *Foramen.*

Ganglion: With respect to the nervous system, a collection of nerve cell bodies located in the peripheral nervous system.

Gray matter: Those regions of the brain and spinal cord, which are made up primarily of the cell bodies and its short extensions (dendrites) of nerve cells. This is in contrast to the longer extensions of the nerve cell that carries electrical impulses (known as white matter or myelinated axons).

Hyperalgesia: Extreme sensitivity to painful stimuli.

Inflammation: A fundamental pathologic process consisting of a dynamic complex of cell and chemical reactions that occur in the affected blood vessels and adjacent tissues in response to an injury or abnormal stimulation caused by a physical, chemical, or biologic agent. The "cardinal signs" of inflammation are redness, heat, swelling, pain, and sometimes inhibited function. They may all be present, but not all are required to be present.

Laminectomy: A surgery to create space by removing some bone (lamina) from the back of the vertebral bone. The resulting decompression can relieve pressure on the spinal cord and nerves.

Magnetic Resonance Imaging (MRI): A diagnostic radiological modality, using nuclear magnetic resonance technology, in which the magnetic nuclei (especially protons) of a patient are aligned in a strong, uniform magnetic field, absorb energy from tuned radiofrequency pulses, and emit radiofrequency signals as their excitation decays. The signals are converted into sets of images by using field gradients in the magnetic field, which permits three-dimensional localization of the point sources of the signals. Unlike CT (conventional radiography) scans or fluoroscopy, MRIs do NOT expose the patient to ionizing radiation.

Naloxone: A potent antagonist or reversal agent of narcotics/opioids. There is no pharmacologic action when administered without narcotics/opioids present.

Narcotic: Any drug, synthetic or naturally occurring, with effects similar to those of opium and opium derivatives, such as morphine and fentanyl. Effects include analgesia (pain relief), mood change, respiratory depression, dependence, tolerance, etc. This term is typically used with respect to law enforcement. The medical field tends to use the word *opioids* to refer to similar drugs.

Nerve conduction study (NCS): This study is usually part of the EMG, which will help test how well signals travel along a nerve. The cause of tingling, numbness, or pain may be assisted by this test. *See Electromyography (EMG).*

Neuroplasticity: The concept that the brain is not fixed, but rather, capable of change or adaptation throughout its lifetime.

Nociceptive: Relating to pain arising from the stimulation of nerve cells.

Nociceptor: Receptor of a sensory neuron (nerve cell) that responds to potentially damaging stimuli by sending signals to the spinal cord and brain.

Noxious: Harmful or unpleasant sensation.

Opiates: Any drug preparation or derivative of opium (e.g., morphine).

Opioids: Term currently used to refer to naturally occurring opiates (e.g., morphine) *and* synthetic narcotics (e.g., fentanyl). Effects include analgesia, mood change, respiratory depression, dependence, tolerance, etc. *See Chapter 8 for more details on Opioids.*

Opioid antagonist: A receptor antagonist that acts on opioid receptors. Typically used as a reversal agent for overdosing on opioids. *See Naloxone as an example.*

Opioid-induced hyperalgesia: A state of making sensory nerves more sensitive to painful stimuli due to exposure to opioids. By weaning down or off opioids, the patient ironically experiences less pain.

Osteopathic philosophy: Philosophy based on four tenets—

- The body is a unit; the person is a unit of body, mind, and spirit.
- The body is capable of self-regulation, self-healing, and health maintenance.
- Structure and function are reciprocally interrelated.
- Rational treatment is based upon an understanding of the basic principles of body unity, self-regulation, and the interrelationship of structure and function.

Osteopathic physician (D.O.): Physicians who are trained to use the diagnostic and therapeutic measures of conventional medicine in addition to manipulative measures, as per the osteopathic philosophy. [In the United States, D.O.s or *osteopathic physicians* are equivalent to M.D.s with respect to their ability to prescribe medication, perform surgery, or specialize in the same fields as M.D.s. In other countries, including Australia, *osteopaths* are typically not physicians but are considered manual medicine experts.]

Osteopenia: Decreased calcification or density of bone, which is a risk factor for osteoporosis.

Osteoporosis: A more advanced stage after osteopenia, whereby bones have become significantly thinner, weaker, and fracture more easily.

Pain: An unpleasant sensory and emotional experience associated with actual or potential tissue damage, or described in terms of such damage.

The extended definition by the International Association for the Study of Pain: "The inability to communicate verbally does not negate the possibility that an individual is experiencing pain and is in need of appropriate pain-relieving treatment. Pain is always subjective. Each individual learns the application of the word through experiences related to injury in early life. Biologists recognize that those stimuli which cause pain are liable to damage tissue. Accordingly, pain is that experience we associate with actual or potential tissue damage. It is unquestionably a sensation in a part or parts of the body, but it is also always unpleasant and therefore also an emotional experience. Experiences which resemble pain but are not unpleasant, e.g., pricking, should not be called pain. Unpleasant abnormal experiences (dysesthesias) may also be pain but are not necessarily so because, subjectively, they may not have the usual sensory qualities of pain. Many people report pain in the absence of tissue damage or any likely pathophysiological cause; usually this happens for psychological reasons. There is usually no way to distinguish their experience from that due to tissue damage if we take the subjective report. If they regard their experience as pain, and if they report it in the same ways as pain caused by tissue damage, it should be accepted as pain. This definition avoids tying pain to the stimulus. Activity induced in the nociceptor and nociceptive pathways by a noxious stimulus is not pain, which is always a psychological state, even though we may well appreciate that pain most often has a proximate physical cause."

Paindemic®: (*Term used by the author*) **The complex epidemic (or pandemic) of chronic pain that persists despite the associated overutilization of pills, injections, and surgeries**. The term implies—

1. The large number of people with pain in the U.S. (and in the world)
2. The epidemic of opioid-related adverse events and overdose deaths in the U.S.
3. The rise of neonatal abstinence syndrome due to pregnant mothers using opioids
4. The enigma of the pain experience itself
5. The lack of education for patients regarding pain's complexity
6. The frustration of contending with an irrational medical system, as in the U.S.
7. The pervasive justification to do riskier and more invasive "treatments" despite lack of strong evidence

Paresthesia: An abnormal sensation such as burning, pricking, tickling, or tingling.

Patient advocate: A person who supports or recommends care or treatment on behalf of what is in the patient's best interest, thereby minimizing risk and maximizing benefit for the patient.

Phantom limb pain: An amputee's experience of pain in the area where the previously existing limb resided. Not all phantom limbs are painful.

Placebo: An inactive substance or treatment given to a patient for its suggestive effect. This can be used in research studies for comparison or in clinical practice just to please a patient. It is believed that the psychological benefit is at play more than the actual physical benefit. This can apply to any noninvasive or invasive approaches for pain.

Plantar fasciosis: A diagnostic term used to explain the heel and plantar fascia pain based on the degeneration of the plantar fascia leading to pain or tightness. This is different than plantar "fasciitis" which is suggesting inflammation.

Plasticity: In human biology terms, it is the *adaptable* or *moldable* ability to change in response to the environment or different lifestyles. Although neuroplasticity is commonly referenced in the medical field, other components of the body (e.g., connective tissue) are also sensing and changing based on various stimuli or input.

Pocket advocate: (*Term used by the author*) A person or entity who supports or recommends care or treatment on behalf of what is most profitable to the business, thereby potentially increasing unnecessary risk despite questionable benefit for the patient.

Postherpetic neuralgia: Pain of a severe, throbbing, or stabbing character along the course of the nerve affected by a herpes virus.

Post-laminectomy syndrome: Presence of back and/or leg pain despite receiving a laminectomy. *Also known as Failed Back Syndrome.*

Radiofrequency ablation: Destruction of a body part, such as a nerve, by using heat.

Referred pain: A complicated phenomena whereby pain is felt to be in an area that is different from the location of the true cause or problem.

Sacrum: The segment of the vertebral column forming part of the pelvis. It closes the pelvic girdle posteriorly or towards the back. It is formed by the fusion of five originally separate sacral vertebrae. It joins the coccyx below, the last lumbar vertebra above, and the hip bones on each side.

Sciatica: A descriptor of pain in the lower back, hip, and especially the back of the thigh. The cause is not obvious by the word sciatica. The symptoms can be caused by direct irritation or pressure on the sciatic nerve by muscle spasms or other connective tissue issues or L5 or S1 nerve root irritation from herniated discs.

Sclerosis: Process by which soft tissues become thickened or hardened.

Self-care: Activities that people do for themselves to establish and maintain health, prevent illness, or cope with illness.

Sensitization: Increased responsiveness or sensitivity of nerves to their normal input, and/or recruitment of a response to smaller inputs. *Central sensitization* refers to changes in the function of neurons within the *central* nervous system only; while *peripheral sensitization* refers to changes in the function of neurons located in the *periphery*, outside the central nervous system. *See Central Sensitization.*

Shingles (herpes zoster): An infection caused by the varicella-zoster virus, the same virus that causes chickenpox. Characterized by an eruption of groups of vesicles on one side of the body following the course of a nerve (dermatome) due to inflammation of the ganglia and dorsal nerve roots. This occurs after reactivation of the virus, which in many instances has remained dormant for years after the initial chickenpox infection. The condition is self-limited but may be accompanied by or followed by severe postherpetic pain.

Spinal stenosis: A painful condition associated with narrowing of one or more areas of the spine. The narrowing can put pressure on the spinal cord or nerves that exit from the spinal column. Symptoms can include severe leg or lower back pain when standing or walking. Leaning over or sitting down tends to relieve the pain. Yet, not all patients with narrowing of their spinal column have pain or neurologic symptoms.

Spondylolisthesis, Lumbar: Forward movement of a lumbar vertebral body on the vertebra below it, or upon the sacrum. There are varying degrees of slippage.

Stellate ganglion: A sympathetic trunk ganglion (cluster of nerve cell bodies) lying behind the large subclavian artery near the origin of the vertebral artery. It is found near the level of the seventh cervical vertebra (C7).

Xanax®: Brand name for alprazolam. *See Benzodiazepines.*

Vertebra: A segment of the spinal column. There are usually 33 vertebrae: 7 cervical, 12 thoracic, 5 lumbar, 5 sacral (fused into one bone, the sacrum), and 4 coccygeal (fused into one bone, the coccyx).

Vertebrae: The plural form of vertebra.

Glossary Sources (if not stated otherwise): Stedman's Medical Dictionary, Merriam-Webster Dictionary, www.Dictionary.com, World Health Organization, International Association for the Study of Pain.

Resources

This is a list of resources, which is merely a place to start on your pain journey. There are many other resources not listed here, which you may find of great value as well. The author does NOT have any financial affiliations with any of these individuals or organizations at the time of printing this book.

Pain Basics:

Educating yourself and reframing your perspective about pain can be incredibly powerful. These can be great overviews of pain as we understand it now. Since any website links can change over time, you can reference the names associated with them to seek further information on your own.

Brief Pain Videos on YouTube, by Neil Pearson, PT, MSc, BA-BPHE, CYT, ERYT500, https://www.youtube.com/user/lifeisnow421/videos

Change Pain®

European website with education and tools for patients and pain professionals

http://www.change-pain.com/

Explain Pain

Book by David Butler and Lorimer Moseley (NOIgroup Publications, 2nd edition, 2013)

Healthskills

Blog site by Bronwyn Thompson

Blog meant for clinicians, but blogs and coping section can be helpful for patients

https://healthskills.wordpress.com/about/

Patient Education Webcast Videos, by Neil Pearson

http://www.canadianpaincoalition.ca/media/video/overcome_pain/part_1/

http://www.canadianpaincoalition.ca/media/video/overcome_pain/part_2/

http://www.canadianpaincoalition.ca/media/video/overcome_pain/part_3/

The Pain Cure Rx: The Yass Method for Diagnosing and Resolving Chronic Pain

Book by Mitchell Yass (Hay House, 2015)

Practical, personalized approach to pain by a physical therapist with extensive experience

Understand Pain Live Well Again

Book by Neil Pearson (ebook available)

"Why Things Hurt" Video, by Lorimer Moseley at TEDxAdelaide (2011)

https://youtu.be/gwd-wLdIHjs

Nutrition:

Focus on more whole foods and fewer processed foods. Here are some guides.

Forks Over Knives

www.forksoverknives.com

Learn Organic Gardening with John Kohler

Entertaining videos

www.growingyourgreens.com

NutritionFacts.org

Short videos and articles on nutrition research

www.nuritionfacts.org

NutritionMD

www.nutritionMD.com

Physicians Committee for Responsible Health

www.pcrm.org/health

Moving and Exercise:

Check with a local gym, personal trainer, or physical therapist to find exercises that are an appropriate progression for you. Daily walking is a low-cost and low-maintenance activity that can be a great goal. If there is inhospitable weather, then you can go online. There are numerous resources and videos for free and for purchase online. Progress slowly to allow every part of your body and brain to adapt with the least chance of injury. Get moving, but move well!

National Health Service Fitness Studio

Free videos. Be aware of what your body is used to doing and modify according to your abilities.

http://www.nhs.uk/conditions/nhs-fitness-studio

Do-It-Yourself Pain Management:

Some ways of managing your pain can be D.I.Y. (do-it-yourself) such as yoga, tai chi, or pilates. Optimizing stability/balance, flexibility, and strength can be achieved through a variety of approaches. The following are some options that can be learned online or in a group. Although they could be taught one-on-one, they tend to be in more of a non-medical setting.

Alexander Technique

Body awareness techniques that can impact pain, balance, and other abilities. Power of habits and intention emphasized with this gentle approach.

www.alexandertechnique.com

Dance Therapy

Individual who overcame pain with dancing

www.dancingwithpain.com

Do-It-Yourself Joint Pain Relief Videos

Gary Crowley has training in Rolfing and other techniques

http://www.do-it-yourself-joint-pain-relief.com/

Feldenkrais®

Gentle movement training and biomechanics awareness

www.feldenkrais.com

Gyrotonic®

Training on equipment with gentle movements

www.gyrotonic.com

The Pain Cure Rx: The Yass Method for Diagnosing and Resolving Chronic Pain

Book by Mitchell Yass (Hay House, 2015)

Mentioned above in pain basics, as it is educational and instructional.

Body Assistants:

When your own efforts or D.I.Y. approaches are not helping, body assistants may be able to help you with better optimization of your body with more pain relief. The extent of the benefit can be affected to varying degrees depending on the option used, the body assistant involved, your body's current state, your body's response, and the consistency of use. Slight improvements over time can lead to significant changes. Pay attention to your body and openly communicate with your health professional(s). And don't forget, your brain is also affected by what you learn and do with your body.

Acupuncturists

Minimally invasive with superficial use of needles

http://mx.nccaom.org/Findapractitioner

Airrosti®

Soft tissue (and joint mobilization) approach to pain.

Emphasis is on intense, short-term treatments with patient self-care education.

www.airrosti.com

Chiropractors

Treatment techniques can vary considerably.

http://www.acatoday.org

Egoscue®

Hands-off postural training focus

www.egoscue.com

Massage Therapists

Treatment techniques can vary considerably.

http://www.ncbtmb.org/tools/find-a-certified-massage-therapist

Osteopathic Manipulative Treatment

Treatment techniques can vary considerably.

http://www.osteopathic.org/osteopathic-health/Pages/find-a-do-search.aspx

Physical Therapists

Treatment techniques can vary considerably.

http://www.apta.org/apta/findapt/index.aspx?navID=10737422525

Selective Functional Movement Assessment (SFMA)

Movement-based diagnostic approach assesses dysfunctional yet non-painful aspects that may be contributing to pain. Techniques to treat the patient can vary based on the specific background of that practitioner.

www.functionalmovement.com

Mindfulness Links:

You can do these in the comfort of your own home or elsewhere. The intention is to be aware and in the moment to calm the nervous system and thereby decrease your pain.

Emotional Freedom Techniques (EFT)/Tapping

Utilizes acupressure points to help some people with pain.

www.emofree.com

Guided Mindfulness Meditation Practices with Jon Kabat-Zinn

www.mindfulnesscds.com

Mindfulness-Based Stress Reduction Program and Resources

Founded by Jon Kabat-Zinn. Based out of the University of Massachusetts

Medical School.
http://www.umassmed.edu/cfm/Stress-Reduction/

Mindful Magazine
www.mindful.org

Online Mindfulness-Based Stress Reduction
Free resources, which include free Jon Kabat-Zinn video links
www.palousemindfulness.com

The Mindfulness Solution
Free meditation downloads
www.mindfulnesssolution.com

Brain Assistants:

Although this is sectioned into "brain," all that you do with your body can affect your brain and vice versa. You can get advice from your primary care physician or other medical professional for resources in your geographic area, but here are some online and in-person options.

American Academy of Pain Management
Psychologists or other professionals can be found at this link
https://members.aapainmanage.org/aapmssa/censsacustlkup.query_page

Beyond Chronic Pain
Coaching service from a therapist with a history of chronic pain
www.beyondchronicpain.com

Goalistics
Online tools developed by two psychologists
http://pain.goalistics.com

Mood Gym Training Program
Online cognitive behavior therapy skills to prevent and treat depression
https://moodgym.anu.edu.au

Post-Traumatic Stress Disorder Coach Online (U.S. Department of Veterans Affairs)
Anyone coping with stress could benefit from this online service
http://www.ptsd.va.gov/apps/ptsdcoachonline

Psychology Today Magazine

Search psychiatrists by zip code and then focus your search to those who treat "chronic pain"

https://psychiatrists.psychologytoday.com

Mobile Pain Log Applications:

There are numerous apps available. Here are two options to note pain trends and recall information better at medical appointments. Yet, overly fixating on pain without focusing on self-care can be counterproductive.

CatchMyPain

www.catchmypain.com

My Pain Diary

www.chronicpainapp.com

Pain Support & Advocacy Groups:

Here are some groups, which may or may not be heavily supported financially by drug, medical device, or other medical industries.

American Chronic Pain Association

www.theacpa.org

Chronic Pain "Meetup" Groups

http://chronicpain.meetup.com/

Pain Action

www.painaction.com

PainPathways Magazine

www.painpathways.org

Power of Pain Foundation

www.powerofpain.org

The National Pain Foundation

www.thenationalpainfoundation.org

The Pain Community

www.paincommunity.org

The Pain Toolkit

www.paintoolkit.org

U.S. Pain Foundation

www.uspainfoundation.org

Specific Condition Support Groups:

Here are only some of the communities with more specific issues in common.

Amputee Coalition of America

www.amputee-coalition.org

Arthritis Foundation

www.arthritis.org

Bridge for Pelvic Pain

www.bridgeforpelvicpain.org

Ehlers-Danlos National Foundation

www.ednf.org

For Grace (*for women in pain, not just CRPS*)

www.forgrace.org

International Adhesions Society

www.adhesions.org

MSWorld (*multiple sclerosis*)

www.msworld.org

National Center for Complementary and Alternative Medicine

www.nccam.nih.gov

National Headache Foundation

www.headaches.org

National Migraine Association

www.migraines.org

National Multiple Sclerosis Society

www.nationalmssociety.org

Reflex Sympathetic Dystrophy (RSD) Syndrome Association

Complex Regional Pain Syndrome (CRPS) replaced the former RSD term

www.rsds.org

Sickle Cell Disease

www.sicklecelldisease.org

The Erythromelalgia Association

www.erythromelalgia.org

Professional Pain Organizations:

These organizations are listed to demonstrate some of the societies of which many pain physicians and other pain providers may be members.

American Academy of Pain Management

Integrative approach emphasized

www.aapainmanage.org

American Academy of Pain Medicine

www.painmed.org

American Board of Anesthesiology

www.theaba.org

American Pain Society

www.ampainsoc.org

American Society of Interventional Pain Physicians

www.asipp.org

American Society of Regional Anesthesia and Pain Medicine

www.asra.com

International Association for the Study of Pain

www.iasp-pain.org

Texas Pain Society

www.texaspain.org

Caregiver-Specific Assistance:

The health of a caregiver or spouse is equally important for the well-being of both parties involved.

Caring Road Support Network

www.caringroad.org

Family Caregiver Alliance
www.caregiver.org
Well Spouse Association
www.wellspouse.org

If you or someone you care about has found other resources helpful, please post that information at www.PainOutLoud.com. Your story and valuable information could help other pain sufferers when you share it with the world.